RETHINKING HEALTHCARE IMPROVEMENT

Philosophy and Ethics in Practice

Alan Cribb, Polly Mitchell and Vikki Entwistle

BLOOMSBURY ACADEMIC
LONDON · NEW YORK · OXFORD · NEW DELHI · SYDNEY

BLOOMSBURY ACADEMIC
Bloomsbury Publishing Plc, 50 Bedford Square, London, WC1B 3DP, UK
Bloomsbury Publishing Inc, 1359 Broadway, New York, NY 10018, USA
Bloomsbury Publishing Ireland, 29 Earlsfort Terrace, Dublin 2, D02 AY28, Ireland

BLOOMSBURY, BLOOMSBURY ACADEMIC and the Diana logo
are trademarks of Bloomsbury Publishing Plc

First published in Great Britain 2026

Cover design by Jade Barnett
Cover image by Susan Wilkinson / Unsplash

A catalogue record for this book is available from the British Library.

A catalog record for this book is available from the Library of Congress.

ISBN: HB: 978-1-350-54712-4
          PB: 978-1-350-54711-7
        ePDF: 978-1-350-54713-1
       eBook: 978-1-350-54714-8

Typeset by Integra Software Services Pvt. Ltd.
Printed and bound in Great Britain

For product safety related questions contact productsafety@bloomsbury.com

To find out more about our authors and books visit www.bloomsbury.com
and sign up for our newsletters.

RETHINKING HEALTHCARE IMPROVEMENT

CONTENTS

ACKNOWLEDGEMENTS

We are very grateful to the many colleagues who have helped us to think about healthcare improvement.

The initial impetus for turning to the questions discussed in this book was Alan's inclusion in the Improvement Science Development Group (ISDG). This created the opportunity to work – in a generous and hospitable setting – with leading improvement researchers from the United States, the UK and Europe. Thank you to ISDG colleagues, not least to Mary Dixon-Woods and Paul Batalden who graciously put time aside to help induct him into this community. Our work in this area, like all healthcare improvement research in the UK, has benefitted substantially from the leadership of the Health Foundation – including their sponsorship and organization of both the ISDG and the Q Community.

The writing of this book was one part of a close and happy collaboration between Alan, Polly and Vikki on a study funded by the Wellcome Trust [209811/Z/17/Z]. The book unquestionably benefitted from other elements of the same project – including key informant interviews with (anonymous) improvement leaders from around the world. We also partnered with a number of invaluable healthcare improvement and research colleagues including Guddi Singh, Alf Collins, Tom Woodcock, Jane O'Hara, Justin Waring, Sharon McCann, Lindsay Oliver, Graham Pullin, Steve Walter, Sonya Crowe and Martin Utley, with whom we co-published articles. We also extend our thanks to Natalie Armstrong, Nick Sevdalis and Craig Ramsay, to members of the Patient and Carer Network of the Royal College of Physicians, and to Jono Broad and Sibylle Erdmann.

In addition, the Wellcome Trust-funded study enabled us to host, and participate in, a considerable range of workshops and events, and we benefitted from listening to many healthcare improvement practitioners, as well as policy makers and fellow academics, in ways that are difficult to trace to individuals.

Both official and unofficial support for the scholarship underpinning this book was kindly volunteered by generous philosophy and bioethics colleagues, including Christian Munthe, Christopher Winch, James Wilson, Lucy Frith, Rob Simpson, Rosamund Scott, Søren Holm, Stacy Carter and Stephen John.

Finally, sincere thanks go to Lucy Harper, the Commissioning Editor for Philosophy at Bloomsbury Academic Publishers, for an encouraging, critically constructive and effective publication experience.

ABBREVIATIONS

AMA	American Medical Association
BMJ	*British Medical Journal*
CQC	Care Quality Commission (England)
IOM	Institute of Medicine (United States of America)
NHS	National Health Service (United Kingdom)
PDSA	Plan–Do–Study–Act
QI	Quality Improvement
RCP	Royal College of Physicians
SDOH	Social Dimensions of Health
UK	United Kingdom
USA	United States of America
WHO	World Health Organization

INTRODUCTION

This book is about the central importance of philosophical questions to healthcare improvement. In it we argue that healthcare improvement – both as a field of study and as action on the ground – should be seen as value-laden, and as an activity that is inherently deliberative and evaluative in an open-ended and qualitative sense. This, we suggest, has important implications for research, education and practice. We imagine that this opening claim will be accepted by many as uncontroversial, but we think the implications are more radical than is generally acknowledged. Our case is not just that attention to deliberation and open-ended evaluation is something to include in the ever-widening knowledge base underpinning improvement work but rather that (a) these things belong at the core of improvement and (b) technical conceptions of evaluation or deliberation are insufficient and that a broadly philosophical engagement with improvement questions is required.

One of our suggestions is that philosophy – the academic field sometimes denoted with a capital *P* – should be treated as one of the 'feeder disciplines' of healthcare improvement, and we hope both to show the relevance of philosophy through the text and to explicitly make a case for the value of that inclusion. But that is perhaps the least far-reaching of our suggestions. More generally we argue that (often small 'p') philosophical considerations and thinking are crucial to the development of a defensible field and practice of improvement. To oversimplify our case, and to put it in very stark, slightly exaggerated, terms that have clear relevance to the field of healthcare improvement, we suggest that healthcare improvement that is disconnected from philosophy is unsafe – that is, potentially dangerous, risky or more liable to cause harms or wrongs to people.

Why are we suggesting this and what are the stepping stones that take us to this conclusion?

First, we argue both (a) that questions about whether something is an improvement are as important, and often as difficult, as questions about how to improve something and (b) that questions about how to improve something, if they are to be tackled responsibly, need to be seen as ethical questions as much as practical-technical ones. In other words, in relation to both purposes and processes, questions about values – how these should be articulated, taken into account, 'weighed' and acted upon – are completely central to improvement. This point is perhaps obvious if we think not just about the specialist domain of healthcare improvement but more simply about how our friends and neighbours would react if we announced we were about to do something to improve their lives.

Second, it is widely understood that improvement efforts may do harm if they are misguided, badly designed or poorly executed. On that basis, healthcare improvement researchers and practitioners will often place importance on both rigorous thinking and conscientious practice.

Third, we argue that the risks attached to improvement often do not have their primary source in the decisions made in relation to specific improvement interventions, but rather arise further upstream, in the way improvement thinking is organized and framed – in the starting points, assumptions, categories, conceptual frameworks and approaches adopted. This entails ensuring that conceptions of rigour and conscientiousness should be extended and applied to the basic framing of improvement thinking and the range of concepts, lenses and practice norms it adopts as well as to the aims and methods being followed in various particular cases.

We hope to show the importance of these philosophical and ethical issues throughout the book, both in general terms and through discussion of examples but here, in summary, we can indicate three linked themes that run through our argument. They all relate to the tendency for healthcare improvement to be seen in technical terms and for improvement knowledge to be seen predominantly as about the development and application of empirical research or 'science'.

The first theme relates to the technical construction of key ideas about what counts as 'success', exemplified in particular by the language of 'quality'. In many instances quality and dimensions of quality (such as effectiveness and safety) are operationalized – i.e. defined and translated into measurements – for research and/or managerial purposes.

Although probably no one would consciously assert that these technical constructions exhaust the meaning of quality ideas, the unintended net effect of operationalization is to conjure a background sense of quality or 'better healthcare' as something that can be understood fully and known concretely. This is a hazard precisely because ideas about quality are contested and unfixed, and there are dangers in inadvertently disguising this contestability with impressions of 'facticity'.

The second theme concerns the limitations of framing expertise about improvement activities in largely empirical terms. An emphasis on understanding causal processes and 'what works' means that it is not only ideas about quality but also characterizations of 'improvement interventions' that are routinely operationalized, with human action often simplified or translated into specified characteristics that can be monitored and measured. This carries two significant risks. First, it fails to capture important aspects of the nature of human action, which is only clumsily represented by more observable features and can only be properly understood in relation to the value-laden purposes and the social fields that shape it. To engage with human action, improvement expertise must extend to an interest in values or, as we will come to label this, be 'normatively conscious'. Second, there are risks of both overestimating and underestimating the role of expert empirical descriptions. As just noted above – in the worry about 'facticity' – technically specified descriptions are overestimated when treated as definitive accounts of reality: they are at best a partial, indicative guide. But they can also be underestimated because to some extent they themselves 'produce facts' and hence create new realities. This is because language and authoritative knowledge are not simply descriptive but also performative and constitutive. ('League tables' of performance provide a familiar example of this – institutions and individuals can question the validity and even meaningfulness of league tables whilst simultaneously taking them seriously and thereby helping to make them matter.)

The third theme relates to the tendency for improvement thinking and action to be undertaken in manageable 'bite-sized' pieces. As with operationalization, there are very good reasons behind this tendency. In different ways both empirical research and practical healthcare planning benefit from drawing parameters and proceeding in defined, relatively focused and local ways. And, certainly, it is impractical to change, or even 'rethink', a whole system all at once. The net result is often an emphasis on finding better ways of 'delivering' prevailing models of good healthcare and good practice, while the complementary (and fuzzier, messier) business of thinking about alternative, more radical, ways of changing healthcare systems and models for the better receives less attention in improvement discourses. The more radical 'revisionary' agendas are, of course, alive and well in other domains. These include debates about the implications of social justice and ecological movements for healthcare, both of which have important implications for conceptions of improvement.

To be clear, we are not suggesting that a technicist delivery-oriented conception of improvement should simply be set aside and replaced with a more open-ended qualitatively evaluative and wholly 'revisionary' conception. The issue is one of balance – we would definitely not, for example, argue that it is intrinsically better or wiser to be more ambitious and disruptive rather than more targeted and conventional in framing improvement. But we do want to stress that people engaged in improvement need to be conscious of the underlying 'choices' embodied in their thinking, and that this means paying attention to the scope of ambition within the field and managing this, as well as other balancing acts and judgement calls, as part of improvement thinking and working.

In other words, moving away from empirical science constructions of research and technicist constructions of practice brings considerable challenges. It involves thinking about how to deal with the recognition that ideas about quality are contested – that there are different dimensions of (and perspectives on) 'better' that need to somehow be acknowledged and handled together and that these dimensions and perspectives can arise and take shape in different contexts for stakeholders with diverse needs and interests. This means that (a) judgements that something is an improvement or that healthcare has become better are likely to be relatively indeterminate, contestable, context-dependent and provisional, and (b) processes of improvement involve managing multiple ethical dilemmas. This is what makes healthcare improvement an inherently deliberative and evaluative domain.

There is, we suggest, an understandable hesitancy to fully embrace the conclusion that judgements about making or evaluating improvements have an indeterminate character. The underlying worry is that the whole enterprise of improvement might effectively collapse because all that is available are 'value judgements' in some pejorative sense – subjective opinions, views and counter-claims – with everything dissolving into relativism. That is why an important part of our ambition in this book is to set out a positive case for embracing 'value judgements' and pluralistic ways of approaching values. This is the reason that philosophy is relevant to improvement and is one of the ways that we aim to bring it to bear on the field. In arguing for this we do not want to overstate the nature of the change entailed. We recognize that there are already broadly 'philosophical' currents in both the academic field and many of the practices of 'improvers' (especially, we think, the latter). One of our hopes is to encourage and to help name and strengthen these existing currents. The title of this book includes 'philosophy and ethics in practice' not only because we are interested in the potential contribution of academic philosophy to the practical field of healthcare improvement but also because we are arguing that the practices of philosophy and ethics are needed and belong in that field.

Who the book is for and how to read it

This book is intended for anyone who has an interest in the quality and improvement of healthcare, an audience which we hope will increasingly include applied philosophers and bioethicists. This is a much bigger group than those who have conscious involvement in healthcare improvement activities, who we will sometimes refer to as 'improvers'. Although it is a somewhat crude shorthand, the term 'improvers' can helpfully cover the loose assembly of agents whose actual or potential activities make up the dedicated field of healthcare improvement, including both professional and lay actors involved in improvement-related healthcare practices, management, leadership, policy, education and scholarship. It is deliberately vague. There is, of course, no presumption that the activities of improvers will always successfully result in improvements. Nor do we assume that everyone in this expansive category will think of themselves under that label – they are likely to apply other labels and to see healthcare improvement as only one of their many concerns.

The book can be read from beginning to end. We have written it with that in mind – structuring it sequentially and developing and elaborating points and adding layers as we go. However, we have also aimed to make the parts and chapters relatively self-sufficient to cater for readers who are interested in particular themes. In places, this means we have erred on the side of repeating key points rather than assuming a reader has attended to earlier chapters. Those who are interested in getting a sense of our case for the relevance of applied philosophy for healthcare improvement should start with this introduction but might also read Chapter 9 where we pull the threads together. In the chapters in-between we both elaborate on our arguments and focus in on specific issues and examples. We hope the summary below and the index will provide a useful guide to people who are interested in specific topics. For example, someone interested in disputes around quality concepts might start with Part 2, or, more specifically, a reader wanting to engage with philosophical complications associated with 'efficiency' will find that in Chapter 4. Likewise, someone with an interest in the opportunities for, and challenges of, expanding conventional constructions of improvement purposes – especially if they are interested in environmental sustainability or anti-racism as emerging priorities – might turn to Chapter 8 first.

The structure of the book

In Chapter 1 we set the scene by introducing healthcare improvement and the possibilities for expansive and critical reflection on and development of it as a field of research and practice. In Chapter 2, we begin to explore some of the complexities involved in making a claim that some change amounts to an improvement. The idea that it is difficult to make justified causal claims about 'what works' in relation to complex systems is acknowledged and relatively well reflected in the field of improvement. What is less widely recognized is that it is equally challenging to make justified normative claims about what matters, whether improvement interventions make things better and whether they should be implemented. We call these phenomena 'explanatory complexity' and 'normative complexity', respectively, and we explore the relationship between them. In brief, we argue that more technicist and empirical claims about improvement are always underpinned, often implicitly, by more open-ended value judgements, and the plausibility of such claims is grounded in specific conceptions of the appropriate aims and function of healthcare. This discussion and, in particular, the idea of 'implicit normativity' are foundational to the argument in rest of the book, as they indicate that conceptual and ethical contestation are deeply embedded in improvement research and practice.

In the remainder of the book, we look much more closely at the range of issues that we have introduced in Part 1. In particular, we consider pluralism and contestability in relation to quality-related concepts (Part 2), the ethical challenges of improvement practices (Part 3) and the potential contributions of philosophy to healthcare improvement (Part 4). We hope to do justice to the way improvement researchers and practitioners are already 'managing' conceptual and ethical questions and also to contribute some further arguments and resources that follow from acknowledging the centrality of these questions and seeking to address them head on. The existing field of healthcare improvement manages the inherently normative nature of improvement in at least two ways. In large part it systematically 'contains' it by placing a technical lens centre stage. But this emphasis is complemented by some strategies that actively consider values and ethical questions.

Part 2 of the book analyses some particularly influential concepts in healthcare improvement by focusing on the idea, and interpretations, of 'quality' and of the various 'dimensions' of quality. The themes introduced in Part 1 about contrasting 'ways of knowing' in healthcare improvement are directly reflected in different understandings and uses of quality concepts such as efficiency, safety, equity and person-centredness. These concepts serve powerful normative functions but are often presented as if they were largely descriptive, seeking to validly represent and measure aspects of healthcare and thereby to provide authoritative and general accounts of 'good' or 'better' healthcare. This is a reductionist move because outside of those technical uses these concepts have varied, indeterminate and contested meanings. Whereas technical operationalization can be useful for certain purposes and is sometimes presented as a 'solution' to open-endedness, we argue that there is also value in embracing relative open-endedness and pluralism with regard to interpretations and judgements of quality. This raises challenges, however, for social coordination and shared action. If improvers cannot unequivocally assess, or agree about, whether something is an improvement – perhaps even along one 'dimension' of quality – how can they proceed?

We look both at seemingly 'harder' concepts such as effectiveness and safety and 'softer' concepts such as person-centredness and equity. Although we go on to problematize this hard/soft distinction, starting with it enables us to raise questions about the role of measurement in improvement, to further investigate some of the tensions between biomedical and social aspects of healthcare improvement, and thereby also to introduce some ethical themes that will be the subject of Part 3. In particular, we note the affinity between a 'harder' framing of improvement which centres on an increase in measured outcomes as success and an 'outcome-oriented' (or 'consequentialist') approach to ethical reasoning. By contrast, we draw out some of the parallels between softer framings of improvement, which highlight multiple overlapping and competing values and conceptions of success, and approaches to ethical reasoning that question the sufficiency of consequentialism.

Part 3 focuses on the ethics of improvement practice and begins our response to the analyses set out in Parts 1 and 2. Recognizing that improvement practices and concepts are plural and saturated in value judgements extends and reconfigures what counts as the ethics of improvement. In the reconfigured version ethics becomes central to every aspect of the field. As we have suggested this entails that some commitment to engage in the analysis of values and ethics (and not only empirical analysis) becomes crucial for the field's pursuit of clarity and rigour. Assumptions or decisions about purposes, descriptive frames and lenses, and improvement approaches and methods, as well as specific actions (at system, organization or service levels) all embody ethical choices and raise ethical questions. These intersecting multiple axes, along with the pluralism arising from diverse perspectives on, and conceptions and dimensions of, quality, make up what we call normative complexity.

Improvement raises ethical questions for practitioners and policymakers about how to proceed in particular cases, but these are also linked into what might be thought of as 'second-order' ethical questions about creating the ethical landscape of healthcare. This is because improvement is, in significant measure, about (or at least aspires to be about) shaping the social conditions of action in health services and policy. In unpacking this idea, we will highlight the 'productive' effects of improvement practices. That is, discourses and activities of improvement create new institutional entities and cultures (most directly as embodied in improvement units and roles) which, in turn, shape health service organizations and values. In other words, the discussion above about technicist ways of studying improvement or interpretations of quality concepts is not just relevant case by case but in creating the kinds of services and climates that people work within.

Given the demanding and complex agenda facing improvement ethics it would be easy for the field of improvement to be overwhelmed by it. The more encouraging news is that healthcare improvement has evolved in ways that already reflect some thoughtful and useful responses to the ethics of improvement. In addition to the work on institutional governance approaches parallel to 'research ethics', there are important substantive practices and procedures designed to reflect and manage normative challenges – for example, to take into account perspectives from diverse stakeholders and to take seriously patient and community values. We suggest that whilst prevailing procedures help to strengthen critical reflection and accountability, they are insufficient and need to be complemented by more self-conscious and philosophical informed approaches to ethical analysis and deliberation.

One concern we anticipate, and take seriously, is the worry that reviewing and unpacking the value contests in healthcare improvement – by focusing more closely on the conceptual and ethical issues in the field – risks doing damage. If all we do is to point to complications and qualifications that provide pervasive grounds for scepticism, we could fall into that trap. Furthermore, given the practical and ethical importance of efforts to improve healthcare this risk extends to indirectly encouraging a serious neglect of healthcare services through the paralysis of thought. And if managing normative complexity requires time-consuming reflection and labour on the part of healthcare practitioners, 'ethical' improvement practice could, in principle, contribute to over-work and staff burnout, and reduce the already-squeezed time available for clinical care and contact with patients. However, we strongly argue, there is no real alternative to acknowledging and attempting to tackle these complexities. Some practical way for improvers to navigate through them, however imperfect, must be found.

Part 4 pulls the narrative threads together, summarizing and highlighting the potential contribution of philosophy and ethics to healthcare improvement. Others have written about the need to 'improve improvement'. How can philosophy help? We present our response in two forms, corresponding with a crude distinction between reconceiving and reinforcing the field of healthcare improvement. We begin by exploring the more 'disruptive' contribution that philosophical perspectives can make. Questioning the field's implicit norms exposes the possibility of 'resetting' the agendas of healthcare improvement. This includes at least two elements. First, it means thinking about more fundamental ways in which the purposes and organizational practices of healthcare might be reworked as, for example, identified in both critical health policy and 'transformation' literatures. This includes calls for a strong switch of emphasis – for example, away from biomedical priorities to some combination of personal well-being or public health priorities. Second, it means opening up greater consideration of some relatively neglected 'dimensions' of quality such as environmental sustainability or anti-racist practice. Exploring the significance of these more 'radical' dimensions, we suggest, also requires some rethinking of approaches and methods, not just aims. These alternative perspectives set localized, technical quality improvement activities, which are often concerned with marginal, closely prescribed gains, within a broader conception of healthcare improvement, which demands consideration of the social value and function of healthcare and the meaning of 'good' healthcare practice. We highlight the social, political and institutional risks of radical reframing, particularly when this moves beyond the theoretical realm and towards practical action.

Finally, we argue that philosophy is particularly well-suited to raise and explore some of the more radical and transformative questions that can, and plausibly should, be asked about improvement. Philosophers are skilled in conceptual and ethical analysis and can adopt what we call a 'trickster role' and an 'insider-outsider stance'. On the one hand, philosophers typically work with a great deal of methodological flexibility, which permits them to ask a surprisingly wide-ranging set of questions and develop answers which don't take a form that would ordinarily be expected in scientific and social scientific disciplines. We particularly emphasize scepticism as a philosophical tool for calling into question accepted beliefs and ideas in improvement research and practice; this promotes reflection on how things might be different, and be thought about differently, and what the implications of this might be. Like a trickster, who questions and subverts the status quo, philosophers can help open up the hermeneutical and transformative possibilities of improvement practice by making space for different understandings and interpretations. Moreover, philosophers typically sit at a critical distance from improvement practice, which allows for the questioning of dominant assumptions and frames in mainstream healthcare improvement and can thereby contribute to the production and analysis of more far-reaching revisionary perspectives. However, the benefits of this 'outsider' perspective only really make sense if coupled with a more 'insider' perspective. That is, philosophers engaging in critical reflection on improvement must do so with knowledge and understanding of improvement practice, rather than with a more abstract representation of what it involves. Without this, it is difficult to see how philosophical critique could be useful to practitioners. Moreover, a more 'bottom-up' approach to philosophical reflection on improvement is needed because philosophical issues recur in different combinations and contexts, and there are few, if any, off the peg answers to complex human and social questions. The right or best thing to do in practice will depend on many empirical considerations and attention to contexts including what is socially feasible. The normatively conscious approach we are proposing is not an alternative to being empirically oriented; rather, it is wholly compatible with, and strengthens, empirical sensitivity.

PART ONE

UNPACKING IMPROVEMENT

1 THE EVOLVING FIELD OF IMPROVEMENT

The improvement of healthcare is probably something everyone thinks about at some point. Given our own healthcare experiences or observations of care given to family members or friends, we make judgements about better and worse care across an indefinitely large range of criteria. We ask: Was the wait too long? Were mistakes made with the medicines prescribed? Did staff show respect and compassion? How could things be improved?

But some people think of healthcare improvement as a field of academic and professional practice. In this latter sense healthcare improvement is an expert field organized around deliberate, systematic, evidence-informed and critically reflective attempts to make healthcare better – albeit a field with fuzzy boundaries and different sub-fields, such as quality improvement, implementation science and improvement studies. There are researchers, clinicians, policymakers and others (including patients and carers) who attend conferences and read journals focused on this field. For some, healthcare improvement is their defining professional identity and specialist role; for others, it is one hat among many. Meanwhile, 'lay people' will often be relatively unaware of this dedicated field and its particularities.

Our aim is to demonstrate the importance of philosophy to healthcare improvement and to invite readers into debates about conceptual and ethical aspects of improvement. This has relevance to both specialist and generalist audiences. Improving healthcare cannot simply be the preserve of some specialist group, and dedicated 'improvers' need, to a substantial extent, to align their concerns and activities with the many others who are interested in improved healthcare.

In the two opening chapters we set the scene. In this chapter, we ask questions about the nature and scope of healthcare improvement and introduce the specialist field. We also start to explore the contrast between a more 'technicist'[1] way of thinking about improvement and more open-ended and expansive ways of thinking about it, which is a thread that runs through the whole book. In the following chapter, we further elaborate this contrast and introduce other themes via an extended example of a healthcare improvement project. The growth of healthcare improvement as a specialism over the past two decades can largely be seen as about drawing on applied sciences to make the field more rigorous. We argue that philosophy has relevance for precisely the same reason. We hope to demonstrate that addressing conceptual and ethical issues in improvement is not an impractical intellectual 'luxury' but a necessary element of making healthcare improvement rigorous and defensible.

Philosophical questions can be asked *about* healthcare improvement (or anything), but we are not primarily interested in analysing the field of healthcare improvement from the outside. Rather, we aim to show how philosophy might contribute *within* the field. Our approach aims to be responsive to the issues facing practitioners working in healthcare contexts. For this reason, we think it is important to start with a summary account of the emergence and characteristics of healthcare improvement as a dedicated field of practice. We are conscious that this diverges from the typical opening of a philosophy book, which might more usually involve a neat statement of a central puzzle. This is a deliberate methodological strategy.[2] We want to situate our philosophical thinking in the untidy, indistinct, political, shifting field of practice – taking it more-or-less as it is, rather than starting from an idealized version of it. Of course, thinking about how healthcare, and healthcare improvement, might be better will involve asking how things could be different in hypothetical and sometimes ideal scenarios. But we suggest that much can be learnt about ideals if we start from the real activities, conventions and concerns of healthcare professionals, patients and researchers.

1.1 Healthcare improvement: A preliminary account

Healthcare improvement is now often seen as a specialist academic-professional field that develops 'sciences of improvement' and applies them through a range of practical methods. It is, however, a field with indistinct boundaries, not least because some of the most compelling exemplars of healthcare improvement took place in the past, and long before a specialist field was recognized and named. One example is Florence Nightingale's work in military hospitals during the Crimean War. Nightingale's overall contributions to healthcare research, environmental health and nursing practice are extensive but include contributions to improving sanitation and safety.[3] Nightingale and the nurses that accompanied her found the sick and wounded soldiers they encountered in awful conditions, with large proportions dying from infectious diseases, often acquired in hospital rather than directly from war wounds. Over several years, during and after the war, based partly on trial and error and increasingly on the analysis of hospital statistics (where she was a pioneer), Nightingale developed her 'Environmental Theory'. This was an account of what is now thought of as 'infection control', setting out the contribution that attention to the quality of air and water and the effective implementation of hand washing and general cleanliness could make to creating safer hospitals. Many of what are now regarded as good hygiene and infection prevention practices – and the institutional and professional standards and guidelines that support them – have their indeterminate roots in historical developments of this kind.

The Nightingale example can illustrate both more narrow and more expansive interpretations of the scope of healthcare improvement. A narrower interpretation might focus on specific 'technologies' or 'improvement interventions', such as initiatives to implement hand washing, and consider the causal contribution that these make to healthcare processes and outcomes. Such consideration would involve looking both at the relevant clinical and social science knowledge base and the practicalities of implementation: do we know that (and ideally why) handwashing is beneficial, do we know what kind of initiatives effectively encourage its widespread adoption and how can we investigate what goes well and/or badly when people try to ensure it happens in various contexts? By contrast, a more expansive interpretation of healthcare improvement might involve thinking about how healthcare has evolved and improved over long periods, and about how various factors have supported this evolution and improvement. Providing good healthcare depends, for example, upon levels and deployment of funding and staffing, service design and organization, professional preparation and continuing education, basic and applied research and technological development, and institutional and occupational regulation. These are influenced by national and global economic, political and social change, wars and other emergencies, and other environmental dynamics. All these factors play a role in the improvement of healthcare and, indeed, will causally interact with specific improvement interventions.

Both narrower and more expansive interpretations are relevant to and sometimes cited in academic summaries of the healthcare improvement field,[4] but the more focused and technical agenda is more typical of work within the specialist field. Nightingale's contribution is significant not only for illustrating the breadth of healthcare improvement, but also as an example of the emergence of a scientific lens on improvement, including the development and use of data collection, representation and analysis, all of which have provided the conditions for the existence of a more narrowly defined healthcare improvement field.

Over the period since the late 1990s, a variety of currents have converged into the notion that healthcare improvement has become, or should aspire to be, a 'science'. Two titles in particular, 'improvement science' and 'implementation science', are now quite widespread. Although the two sub-fields they refer to are increasingly seen as strongly overlapping or convergent, they arise from two complementary traditions and problem-sets.[5]

Improvement science has its roots in the industrial context and the management of 'quality' in manufacturing. Quality improvement (QI) practices were developed on industrial production lines early in the twentieth century to help monitor and prevent or, failing that, filter out defective goods or those which fail to conform to specifications, which were a sign of waste as well as a source of unsatisfactory experience or harm to consumers. QI methods were subsequently adopted and adapted to improve health services. The simplest, most longstanding and still very influential model used to guide improvement on the ground is PDSA (or Plan–Do–Study–Act). This is a cycle in which desired improvements are specified, then improvement-oriented actions introduced in small-scale ways with data collected and analysed before and afterwards to review their effects, leading to further rounds of planning and action to roll out, refine and monitor change. The PDSA model is indicative of the way that improvement methods typically knit together practice and research or reflection. Critics of the QI approach sometimes comment that healthcare is different from industrial manufacturing and that healthcare is not a factory. This is an important observation, but some aspects of healthcare are factory-like, at least in some respects, and the parallels create scope for healthcare to benefit from methods designed to prevent or fix industrial production or performance failures.

Whereas improvement science has its roots in the problem of performance failures, implementation science has its roots in the problem of unproductive or 'idle' knowledge. Implementation science is typically associated with the rise of the evidence-based medicine movement. This movement has emphasized the need to test the effectiveness of medical treatments and other healthcare interventions empirically rather than assume they work because there is a plausible theory of how they work or because they are recommended by a respected authority.[6] It encourages weeding out treatments that are demonstrably ineffective and using the best available knowledge from clinical epidemiological research (typically large, well-designed, randomized controlled trials comparing the effects of different interventions in practice, and systematic reviews of the results of these trials) to guide practice. Recognition that the uptake of interventions that had been positively evaluated via such research was often slow and patchy led to questions about how knowledge from research could be translated into practice and how demonstrably effective interventions could be spread across institutions and systems. The organizing idea of implementation science is that efforts to spread evidence-based practices and bring about service and system change also need to be informed by systematic research and well-tested theory. Implementation science work has built upon longstanding studies of 'knowledge utilization' and 'policy implementation' including, for example, the tradition of work on 'diffusion of innovations' from the first half of the twentieth century.[7]

As the healthcare improvement field has evolved, recognition has been given to an increasingly large set of improvement 'methods', including the collation and curation of these into overviews and guides. For example, the Healthcare Quality Improvement Partnership's guide to quality improvement introduces and explains twelve methods (including PDSA, Lean/Six Sigma, Statistical process control and Root cause analysis) suited for a range of different purposes.[8] The 'Improvement Method Olympics', a 2021 Twitter competition organized by NHS Horizons, which served as a gentle educational overview of the field, included thirty-two distinct methods that voters could rank according to value.[9] As that competition made clear the term 'methods' is sometimes used in a very broad way, ranging from relatively simple tools to more complex overarching approaches. It includes a variety of 'templates', 'protocols' or 'practical frameworks' intended to support a systematic approach to improvement. Improvement 'methods' are about '*how*' to practise improvement. They crystallize practical improvement 'know-how' into words and diagrams that offer common reference points, which can be shared within and across teams and used to help plan and steer improvement activities. Implementation sciences have also developed a range of practice-oriented frameworks that help guide planning and action including possible strategies and steps, potential enablers and barriers to improvement, and approaches to evaluation. Some of these have been synthesized into higher-level models, meta-protocols and principles for improvement work.[10] The surface features of many such 'methods' – designed as they are to provide relatively simple overview starting points – disguise the complexity faced by improvement practitioners and the sophistication and reflectiveness of debates around both models and practice, as elaborated in the associated academic literature.

Together the two interlinked currents of improvement and implementation science, in combination with the practices they stimulate and support on the ground, provide an indicative sketch of what we are calling the specialist field of healthcare improvement. But we will not stipulate any rigid boundaries around this field. In the way we are using it, improvement typically involves deliberate and systematic efforts to change the organization or culture of care within or across institutional settings. That is, we are largely excluding some kinds of activities, such as those that contribute to healthcare improvement indirectly or accidentally, or very small-scale cases where individuals, but not necessarily services, may 'improve' in some respects (e.g. individual health professionals undergoing training to enhance their knowledge and skills). In what follows we interpret 'improvement activities' in a very expansive sense that encompasses (at least):

1   Practices of improvement including

   - making judgements about potential 'shortfalls' in care quality, or other positive opportunities to strengthen provision;

   - enacting 'improvement interventions' designed to improve healthcare;

   - monitoring, measuring or otherwise evaluating the effects of interventions and approaches.

2 The development of 'improvement practice knowledge' – including local, informal forms of knowledge and evidence from clinical audits and epidemiological sciences – that inform, or form the knowledge base for, healthcare improvement practices.

3 Broader educational, research and scholarly activities directed towards understanding and supporting the field of healthcare quality and improvement.

1.2 The relevance of philosophy

How is philosophy relevant to the complex and historically situated set of activities and institutions that make up the field of healthcare improvement? In this and the following section we start to sketch an answer to this question.

A concern with understanding how practices and institutions can be better or worse is a relatively familiar concern in philosophy, albeit not one usually addressed under the label of 'improvement'. Rather, philosophers have typically considered questions we might associate with improvement with an ethical idiom in the foreground. In political philosophy, for example, it has long been a mainstream concern to ask on what basis institutions might be designed and arranged to better support valuable ends, such as fairness, social justice, or to optimize the chance of everyone having their needs met.[11] Similarly, both ancient and more contemporary philosophers have encouraged us to think about how individuals can cultivate and achieve various virtues and 'excellences' and how social institutions and practices might be organized to support such excellences,[12] including the particular kinds of goods that are 'internal' to practices (e.g. 'care' in health and social care, or 'learning' in educational settings).[13] More broadly, there is very extensive debate in philosophical ethics about concepts such as 'good' and 'bad', 'right' and 'wrong', and the relationships between them.

Thus, although the idea and field of practice of 'healthcare improvement' may feel unfamiliar to philosophers, many of the conceptual and ethical questions they raise mimic those that arise whenever philosophers think about social institutions and complex human activities and practices. There are conceptual questions to be addressed about what the core ideas and commitments within a field mean, and whether they are defined and used in coherent and justifiable ways. There are questions about what count as relevant forms of expertise and capability and whether and where these exist. And there are questions about theoretical and practical ethics, which might consider, for example, what goods and values institutions – including healthcare institutions – ought to pursue and by what means they ought to strive towards them or how different actors should conduct themselves in practice, including in balancing competing values and priorities and making decisions that are ethical, in both their means and ends.

While there are many possible starting points for philosophical engagement in healthcare improvement, we begin here with the central question of how to identify some change as an 'improvement'. Within the context of philosophical discussion, the idea of making things 'better' opens a range of debates about what counts as better and why. People's contrasting and sometimes rival perspectives and interests lead them to operate with competing conceptions of 'better', and there are philosophical questions and disputes about how determinations about what is 'better' can and should be made. Almost by definition any claim that something is better will have value contests and uncertainty close to its core.

We can ask, in relation to any putative improvement: Why is that better? How should we go about making such judgements? As discussed in the previous section the mainstream field of healthcare improvement often draws on the language of 'science', and the question of what counts as an improvement is typically dealt with in a neutral-seeming technical idiom.[14] In other words, judgements about what is or would be better are often approached in large measure as empirical questions, or as matters of fact. But this sort of judgement is not purely about facts. Even within a technical context, for these exercises to make sense, some kind of evaluation (some application of value judgements) must be taking place – criteria or standards that are deemed to be relevant to judging something as better are being adopted and applied, and observations or other data are assessed against this to inform conclusions. Outside of a technical context the question about what counts as better will very often be seen primarily as a question about weighing values and value judgements. Two people disagreeing about which of their local health clinics is better, or which of two political parties has the better vision for the health system as whole, may not disagree significantly about the features of those clinics or systems that are typically presented as facts. Rather they may place stress on different values and make different judgements as a result. In both the technical and non-technical cases, evaluation is happening, but the evaluation process looks rather different. In the technical case something like a template is specified or assumed and the relevant data compared against it. The judgement criteria that are built into the template are value-laden, but this tends to be forgotten because of the technical emphasis. In the non-technical case what is at stake is precisely what kind of criteria are relevant and how they should best be interpreted and applied.[15] These two forms of evaluation are linked: the specification of what is important in the technical setting inevitably raises questions about where these value criteria come from and why they represent what would be good or better, that is, it raises more open-ended normative questions that cannot be answered in technical terms. In addition to healthcare improvement resting on conceptions, both explicit and implicit, of what counts as better it is also fuelled by an ethical imperative which tends to be unspoken but surfaces from time to time. This imperative features most obviously in justifications for the field: healthcare policies and services can make people's lives better or worse in substantial respects and in diverse ways, and improvements reduce the chance of bad things happening and/or make good things more likely. Healthcare improvement thus links technical and ethical concerns. If we want to reason well about it, we need to study both sets of concerns at the same time and ensure that they are connected.

The importance of attending to both facts and values when thinking about the nature and justifiability of complex social institutions is by no means a new idea: this is the basis of much applied ethics, including healthcare and health policy ethics. However, the prevalence of technicist thinking in the healthcare improvement context, which tends to obscure the value judgements (or 'normativity') in play, provides a good reason for spelling out and emphasizing this thought. Recognizing the normative and contested nature of claims about what is better is an important first step to thinking critically about improvement as a practice.

Starting from the challenge 'But why is that better?' opens up a whole host of other philosophical and ethical issues. It raises conceptual questions about the definitions of good healthcare and its component parts, broad ethical questions about the appropriate values to promote and pursue in healthcare, and a wide range of more specific practical-ethical and epistemic challenges. For example, what is the relative importance of different values in healthcare and how should they be balanced against one another? How should variation and disagreement about the meaning and priority of healthcare values be managed? To what extent, if at all, should social values which are not directly related to healthcare be considered? Should, and how far should, attempts be made to resolve difference and standardize definitions? In practice, how can claims of improvement be substantiated and evidenced, given normative disagreement? To what extent should improvers be thinking about the means as well as the ends of improvement activities? How far, in temporal, geographical and institutional terms, should improvers be expected to look for the effects of improvement activities? That is, asking questions about what counts as 'better' and why highlights a whole range of ways that technicist emphases within the field of improvement are open to challenge. Addressing, or at least recognizing, conceptual and normative ambiguities and assumptions that underpin improvement practices and claims about healthcare improvement is a central part of addressing the justifiability of such practices and claims.

One can be more or less rigorous in attending to and characterizing both facts and values. There is much discussion of rigour, and how to enact competing conceptions and approaches to it, in the empirical sciences, including improvement and implementation sciences. Something analogous applies in normative reasoning. Value conflicts and contested evaluations need not be seen as merely reflecting contradictory personal opinions about which nothing more can be said. Rather, interlocutors can acknowledge, identify and clarify the values that underpin their thinking and set out what they propose are crucially relevant arguments and kinds of evidence to elucidate and defend their conclusions. And value divergence can reflect the different social and institutional perspectives occupied by different people – differences which are highly salient to thinking about improvement priorities. Importantly, evaluation can fail to involve such normative reflection and overlook potential value conflicts and areas of contestation. Both descriptive and normative justifications need to be considered to assess the rigour of claims about improvement.

The distinction we are making between technical and non-technical faces of evaluation – with the latter positively 'inviting in' debate about values – does not only apply to judgements about what is 'better' but also to judgements about what counts as 'shortfalls' in healthcare, to which we turn next.

1.3 Two ways of thinking about what is wrong with healthcare

The motivation for improving healthcare might be condensed into the idea that there is something wrong, or at least suboptimal, with healthcare that should be corrected. As just noted, this can be seen, at least in part, as an ethical concern. We can distinguish between two main ways in which something might be thought to be wrong: first, when healthcare falls short on its own terms and, second, when problems are identified with the terms on which healthcare operates. In the first set, roughly speaking, ethical shortcomings derive from technical shortcomings – because what was promised or expected has not been delivered. Healthcare improvement as a field has historically been focused on such technical shortcomings and often adopts what we will refer to as a 'delivery' perspective. In the second set, the expectations, norms and models adopted within healthcare are themselves the subject of critique or revision because what is promised or expected is thought to be misguided in some respects. Healthcare improvement has traditionally been less concerned with these more open-ended ethical concerns which contribute to what we call a 'revisionary' perspective. A revisionary perspective is perhaps closer to the core of related fields such as healthcare ethics and sociology of health where healthcare norms routinely come under analytical and critical scrutiny. The distinction between delivery and revisionary perspectives is meant to be somewhat crude: both perspectives co-exist in the field and the two come together in various ways. But the distinction helps to expose some of the limitations of ways of thinking about healthcare improvement which (often implicitly) treat some of the more revisionary concerns as out of scope. We will consider the delivery and the revisionary emphases in turn.

1.3.1 A delivery perspective

The field of healthcare improvement is substantially motivated by the aspiration to close the gap between what can reasonably be hoped to happen if health services work as intended and what actually happens. It is, to a large extent, driven by these 'delivery' questions, centrally including: are less effective treatments being used when more effective treatments exist? Is there waste of resources and efforts within systems and processes? Is the way people are being treated (or not treated) by health services causing avoidable harm? To identify and address such issues, improvers engage with challenges around logistics, the management of technology, audit and quality assurance, service design and coordination, staffing, behaviour change, teamwork and peer learning, institutional and system leadership and so on. It is not easy to meet any one of these challenges, let alone to address them all together.

An influential version of this delivery perspective, and of the need for systematic attention to healthcare improvement, was set out in the Institute of Medicine's 2001 report on US healthcare services, *Crossing the Quality Chasm: A New Health System for the 21st Century*. The executive summary of this now classic document states:

> Health care today harms too frequently and routinely fails to deliver its potential benefit. Americans should be able to count on receiving care that meets their needs and is based on the best scientific knowledge. Yet there is strong evidence that this frequently is not the case.[16]

The scale of the problem is set out in stark terms:

> tens of thousands of Americans die each year from errors in their care, and hundreds of thousands suffer or barely escape from nonfatal injuries that a truly high-quality care system would largely prevent [...] [Safety] reflects only a small part of the unfolding story of quality in American health care. Other defects are even more widespread and, taken together, detract still further from the health, functioning, dignity, comfort, satisfaction, and resources of Americans.[17]

Crossing the Quality Chasm offers an analysis of some of the reasons health services can fall short. Prominent amongst these is the fact that both the tools and agendas of healthcare are constantly evolving. If the best scientific knowledge is going to be applied this means somehow translating the ongoing development of research and technical innovation in ways that can be incorporated into workable and steadily evolving institutional and professional routines. Overlapping with this, the report highlights both epidemiological and cultural changes that bring new demands for health services in countries like the United States. The broad trend towards increased life expectancy (albeit a trend that is now faltering in some contexts) and the increasing prevalence of chronic illness increase demand on care resources and already at the time of the report represented the largest element of healthcare expenditure. Rising levels of chronic illness also require the development and implementation of new models of care – with partnerships between professionals and patients being a key component for managing conditions that are mainly experienced and dealt with by the people who live with them at a distance from clinical spaces. The report highlights two other causes of the partial failure of health services – a 'poorly organized delivery system' and the limited harnessing of the then comparatively recent 'revolution in information technology'.[18] According to the report's authors the health system under description at that time was not merely unsuited to providing the level of coordination required for the rise of chronic illness but was inherently fragmented and over-complicated:

> less like a system than a confusing, expensive, unreliable, and often impersonal disarray ... Care delivery processes are often overly complex, requiring steps and handoffs that slow down the care process and decrease rather than improve safety.[19]

Based on this account of patients and clinicians experiencing high levels of frustration as services fall short of delivering consistently high-quality services, the report makes strategic recommendations and calls for substantial action and change not only to address prevailing quality deficits but to reorient services by addressing what it calls six 'improvement aims':

Healthcare should be:

- *Safe* – avoiding injuries to patients from the care that is intended to help them.

- *Effective* – providing services based on scientific knowledge to all who could benefit and refraining from providing services to those not likely to benefit (avoiding underuse and overuse, respectively).

- *Patient-centred* – providing care that is respectful of and responsive to individual patient preferences, needs and values and ensuring that patient values guide all clinical decisions.

- *Timely* – reducing waits and sometimes harmful delays for both those who receive and those who give care.

- *Efficient* – avoiding waste, including waste of equipment, supplies, ideas and energy.

- *Equitable* – providing care that does not vary in quality because of personal characteristics such as gender, ethnicity, geographic location and socioeconomic status.[20]

Although *Crossing the Quality Chasm* was written over twenty years ago, and for the US context, its main contours – including its account of challenges facing health services and the ways they can fall short – have retained their relevance for many broadly comparable health systems. Discussions of healthcare improvement often begin with justifications that highlight shortcomings in safety and uneven, often poor, healthcare delivery as core concerns. For example, jumping forward almost twenty years, Mary Dixon-Woods, Founding Director of The Healthcare Improvement Studies Institute, began a *BMJ* essay about healthcare improvement in the context of the UK NHS with the same central emphasis: 'In the NHS, as in health systems worldwide, patients are exposed to risks of avoidable harm and unwarranted variations in quality.'[21]

This core case for improvement has now been reiterated by policymakers, professionals, specialist agencies and others countless times, and the underlying sense of healthcare improvement as an ethical imperative has been further fuelled by a series of scandals in which concentrations of poor care – within specific institutions or in relation to specific groups of patients – have been put under the spotlight. Dixon-Woods continues her essay:

> The National Confidential Enquiry into Patient Outcome and Death, for example, has raised many of the same concerns in report after report. Catastrophic degradations of organisations and units have recurred throughout the history of the NHS, with depressingly similar features each time.[22]

The delivery perspective reflected in these accounts is undoubtedly very important to identifying and understanding problems and designing and delivering well-functioning health services. But, particularly when issues of patient safety or gross malpractice are emphasized, it is easy to characterize the ethical issues that arise in relation to delivery gaps too simplistically – as cases of bad things happening which could and should have been straightforwardly stopped or prevented. In practice, delivering good healthcare is typically far more complicated and interesting, and requires the kinds of balancing of commitments and priorities that will be familiar to those with an interest in priority setting and resource distribution. Given a range of improvement aims and finite, if to some extent flexible, resources, decisions will have to be made about how to prioritize and balance desired outcomes of and ambitions for changes to services. There are questions to be considered about how the different aims interact: Are some lexically prior to others, such that no gains in relation to one aim, no matter how large, can justify any decrease in a lexically prior aim? Or are trade-offs between all aims permissible, and if so, with what caveats or guidance? Even if there were resources to support all desired improvement projects – an unlikely prospect in most actual or feasible healthcare systems – some priority setting will be needed, as decisions will have to be made about what to pursue first. These are practical questions with crucial ethical components, for they require reasoning about values and their relative status – thinking about the range of things that matter and how urgent and important they are. Aside from these questions about how the values in question relate to one another, there are more substantive questions about the meaning and implications of the stated aims of healthcare which are more-or-less taken as given within a 'delivery' perspective. These include practical-conceptual questions about what 'safe' or 'effective' or 'equitable' care requires in practice, as well as epistemic questions about what standards and measures can and should be used to make justified assessments about 'safety', 'effectiveness', 'equity' and so on. We discuss these issues further in Part 2 of the book.

Adopting a delivery perspective on improvement can implicitly assume that the values guiding health service delivery are on the whole the right ones, even though improvements need to be made in some areas. But sometimes, clear and definitive statements of systemic aims and performance gaps can miss other ways of thinking about how things might go wrong with health systems and healthcare improvement. Questions might reasonably arise, for example, about whether the stated aims of healthcare improvement miss out important elements. Or whether the explicit priorities of healthcare systems really capture their most important aspects or attributes, or whether some core values have been left out or are downplayed (e.g. by being definitionally subsumed under another value). Alternative definitions of values or alternative sets of values might, for example, be favoured by groups of people with particular experiences, perhaps reflecting their professional, patient or other socially significant identity characteristics. Addressing this further set of issues is crucial for understanding the nature and significance of delivery gaps, but it also seems to raise more fundamental or open-ended questions about what matters and about how to choose between different and potentially broader visions of what health systems should hope to achieve and promote.

1.3.2 A revisionary perspective

There have, of course, been changes over the more than twenty years since *Crossing the Quality Chasm*. For a start, as indicated above, the language and the field of healthcare improvement, including QI tools and implementation strategies, have become mainstream features of health systems, research and policy. In addition, there has been an expansion in broader improvement-related discourses. First, the widespread acceptance and visibility of the need to improve the 'delivery system' of healthcare has coincided with an increasing expectation that patient groups, members of the public and the media, as well as policymakers and managers, can and should be able to subject health services to critical scrutiny. Second, the range of concerns commonly articulated in the public domain has grown. To some extent this expanding agenda is already anticipated in the IOM's 'six aims' listed above and in the report's discussion of the need for new models of care.

The IOM's aims arguably incorporate at least a partly 'revisionary' lens into the official improvement agenda. The prominent inclusion of patient-centredness as an aim of healthcare was relatively novel at the time and, while it has gained traction in the past two decades, concerns about whether healthcare is 'patient-centred' (or these days more often 'person-centred') raise questions that challenge and go far beyond logistical, operational or delivery challenges. The aim of equity similarly raises questions about what healthcare systems services ought to do, look like and feel like. One way of characterizing the shift of emphasis from a delivery to a revisionary perspective is to say that an aim like 'patient-centredness' or 'equity' might start off by being used in a largely descriptive sense – capturing one aspect of what is already regarded as good practice (e.g. the idea that it includes being responsive to patient values or ensuring the same level of quality for all people using a service) but that articulating and taking seriously this idea then stimulates more radical questions about values: What (range of things) might being responsive to patient values entail? What would constitute equal or equitable responsiveness across diverse patient groups, and can this be achieved within current healthcare and health system practices?

A revisionary perspective on improvement reflects a different, albeit complementary, conception of 'falling short' or 'failing' than a delivery perspective. As indicated earlier we can perfectly well decide that a health service practice is functioning exactly as intended but that it nonetheless ought to be changed. Calls for new 'models of care' – for example, to improve the management of chronic illness – can be based on a delivery-perspective recognition that health service effectiveness requires the application of new ways of working to apply existing standards and expectations to evolving challenges or to incorporate new technologies. But such calls can also spring from judgements that some existing expectations are ethically inadequate or plain wrong – that current standards or models of practice are, to varying degrees, lacking compassion, disrespectful, insensitive, unresponsive, mis-targeted, discriminatory, or otherwise unequal or unfair. Again, there is significant overlap with a delivery perspective here. A key part of what makes healthcare failures into scandals is that they provide evidence of actual named people being neglected and their concerns and needs not being seen or met. But there are many other cases where the 'ethical shortfall' is potentially equally serious but less obvious, more contestable and where the 'victims' and harms are more difficult to discern, for example because lesser service responsiveness to the needs of some groups of patients is relatively subtle and outcome distribution patterns are hard to recognize and attribute to healthcare causes. One important set of factors underpinning actual or possible 'ethical shortfalls' is that just as demographic and illness patterns have evolved, so have social values and norms.

Much of the discussion and analysis of shortfalls in the prevalent standards or expectations of healthcare takes place outside of the fields of healthcare improvement or health services research. It is more often found in disciplinary areas such as sociology of health, radical social policy or healthcare ethics, or within critical social movements or patient advocacy organizations. There are also many examples and parallels to be found in the broader public culture in an age where professional paternalism and associated language, such as that of patient 'compliance', are often seen as inappropriate and frequently contested. But – as we will discuss in the following section – mainstream thinking about the limitations of health services increasingly resonates with, and is influenced by, many of these sceptical and critical currents, especially those rooted in worries about various forms of inequality including the distribution of power within health systems and relationships, the importance of recognizing diverse identities and voices and the (typically unintended) differential effects of health systems on sub-populations and groups.

Illustrative examples of worries about how health services might 'go wrong' because they are inappropriately oriented or working to models and standards that neglect key value concerns include:

- Relative neglect of the social determinants of health: Health services, in the way they are organized or enacted, might not pay sufficient attention to the 'upstream' factors that produce poor health and/or inequalities in health experiences instead focusing on delivering treatments or interventions 'downstream'. Downstream interventions may be relatively ineffective because the more deep-seated causal factors continue to operate.

- Failure to contain or restrict 'medicalization': Health services may provide and indirectly promote biomedical and institution-focused answers for people's problems when there might be 'better' (more effective, empowering and engaging) alternatives which are more social and psychosocial in character.

- Absence of 'co-production' of services: Services may fail to meaningfully engage with, or reflect the values, preferences and capabilities of, the people and communities they are meant to serve.

- Lack of recognition, or tackling, of structural biases including micro-aggressions: Groups of people may be relatively neglected or treated in damaging ways within services because of institutional discrimination or conscious and unconscious bias.

All these kinds of harms and wrongs can be fostered by the structures and cultures of health service organizations; addressing them requires action at an institutional or system level rather than solely through the good intentions and practices of individual actors.

It is, however, worth noting that it is often easier to specify bad healthcare than good healthcare. If a treatment is used inappropriately and causes needless suffering to people, then likely everyone will agree that this is a bad thing. But the same people may not agree about what would count as the right thing to do in the same situation, especially if we allow them an 'aspirational' lens on healthcare which permits them to think about what they would see as ideal, and not just adequately good, healthcare.

The historically dominant framing of healthcare improvement centres on 'closing the delivery gap'. But we have also noted that the overall agenda of improvement – even understood as a circumscribed field of practice and research – is broader than that. Thinking about what might be entailed by a revisionary perspective thus highlights two axes relevant to all improvement activities. Crudely speaking we might see the first axis as a 'vertical' one ranging from very bad to very good (with a threshold of 'adequately good' somewhere in between), i.e. delivering 'good care' is not the only possible ambition. In addition, as the six aims from *Crossing the Quality Chasm* already indicate, there are also multiple respects in which healthcare can be better or worse. So the second crude axis would be a horizontal one representing the diverse ways that healthcare could be relatively good or bad. The horizontal axis may call for different kinds of thinking depending on the kinds of 'goods' and 'bads' in question, and this can complicate or challenge the delivery framing. For example, both person-centred care and equity can mean a range of things, and it is not necessarily useful to close down this variety (we will come back to this in Chapter 5). Person-centred care includes acknowledging that what counts as good care can vary from person to person and has a cultural dimension, and that healthcare is not just about providing things to people but is about relating to them and doing things with them. This has the potential to pose serious challenges to the presumed value of standardization and problem of postcode lotteries, which are often central to delivery perspectives on improvement. Similarly, there is no stable or agreed way of characterizing equity in healthcare. Taking equity seriously opens up extremely complex questions about how and when to respond to different kinds of needs, expectations and identities including questions about historical treatment, recognition, participation or distribution of resources[23] – factors that can pull policy and practice in conflicting directions.

One of the themes that we develop and discuss across the book is how the framings that are implicit in the way people think about and enact improvement practices are critically important. The assumptions that precede discussion and action determine such a lot of what is thereafter thought to matter, including how progress is evaluated. One example of this is the influence of a strong delivery perspective on improvement discourses. There is at least a danger, we suggest, that a dominant 'delivery' framing may obscure or distort improvement thinking – or at least limit its scope substantially – unless other, more revisionary, conceptions of what could count as healthcare falling short or being improved are somehow kept in mind.

1.4 The expanding agenda and field of healthcare improvement

There are at least two linked respects in which attention to healthcare improvement might be said to have expanded since the 1990s. First, the social and cultural context of healthcare has changed and this, as just noted in relation to the growth of revisionary perspectives, includes widespread discussion and debate – far beyond the specialist field – about the purposes and quality of healthcare and health policies. Second, the specialist field of healthcare improvement has grown along with the repertoire of approaches, methods and organizing frameworks. The scholarly agenda for, and disciplinary base of, improvement has expanded, reflecting the existence of multiple perspectives on improvement, including an increasing range of academic, as well as (sometimes connected) community-based, contributions. These changes mark a shift – that we are welcoming and hoping to contribute to in this book – towards a more self-consciously value-laden and open-ended conception of healthcare improvement. Philosophical analysis has the potential to interrogate and further develop this expansive conception of improvement, in part by exploring foundational questions and more fundamental revisionary possibilities.

The decreasing acceptability of medical 'paternalism' from the 1960s on, in the UK, the United States and many other countries, is a high-profile example of ongoing social change. It highlights how conceptions of good healthcare evolve because of cultural as well as technological change, and it makes some of the previously obscured normative underpinnings of healthcare visible. The idea that clinicians should behave prescriptively and authoritatively, and in so doing perhaps choose not to share information about diagnoses, prognoses or treatment options with patients, is nowadays rejected on a widespread basis. Norms have shifted such that there is now a standard expectation that not only all key information but also many key decisions are shared with patients. Translating the implications of these shifts for practice is a continuing challenge. But this is just one facet of a much broader constellation of changes to social relationships and power dynamics. These include changes to the place of professional groups in society and to professional norms. Although it varies from country to country there have been general policy trends that effectively qualify the social power of professional groups, including the medical profession, by, for instance, subjecting professions to combinations of market (or quasi-market) and managerial forces. These trends – because, for example, they mobilize institutional competition or comparison and discourses of 'patient choice' – partly overlap with a wider rise in public scrutiny including from patient advocacy groups, health-related social movements and other critical voices in traditional and new media. To a large extent these broad shifts have also been reflected, incorporated and often welcomed *within* professional practice. For example, the increasing aspiration for 'shared decision-making' can be seen as symbolic of the broader rise in discourses of partnership and collaboration. This includes the rise of inter-professional working which redraws or refines some of the hierarchies between professional groups, increasing calls for 'co-production' with patients in service design and policymaking, and increased sensitivity to differential experiences of people with diverse identities and cultural norms. These changes have also encountered critical scrutiny: Is there a risk of devaluing medical expertise and knowledge and over-valuing personal tastes and preferences? Does the decline of a highly protected professional sphere in healthcare risk empowering commercial actors, backed by advertising campaigns and representing corporate interests, rather than patients? And to what extent should it be concerning if measures to promote population health are compromised by a shift towards patient choice and emphasis on autonomy?

This broad constellation of changes has inevitably brought some normative discussion and ethical questioning into conversations about what counts as better healthcare and is clearly relevant for thinking about healthcare improvement. It is not merely that anyone interested in improving healthcare needs to take into account an enlarged set of expectations and constituencies. It also means that at least some of the focus of healthcare improvement must shift to accommodate evolving, and sometimes contested, norms. These norms are relevant not merely as part of the backcloth to healthcare improvement but as part of its substance. There will always be aspects of judging what counts as better healthcare that depend critically upon clinical expertise but there will be other aspects – including those about care relationships, communication and inclusion – that depend upon value debates and more diffuse forms of knowledge. It may not be possible to settle on a single, clear answer about the appropriate balance and distribution of different values and goods, because of the wide range of healthcare contexts and perspectives which any healthcare system incorporates. Healthcare improvement must manage a good deal of uncertainty, including value uncertainty, in making claims about and making efforts to bring about better healthcare.

Over the first twenty-five years of this century, healthcare improvement as a field of practice and study has also expanded and evolved. As we write in 2025, improvement-related practices and discourses are pervasive in policy, health services and academic contexts. There are now established national and international agencies and networks focused on healthcare improvement. In some national contexts, such as the UK, very many larger health-service organizations have established dedicated improvement teams to work in partnership with front-line teams of 'improvers' (as well as Boards and other service leaders). In addition, healthcare improvement research activity, judged by volume, including the proliferation of academic journal titles, has substantially increased over the last twenty-five years.[24] The consolidation and development of a stronger institutional locus for the field have been accompanied by a growth in the range of approaches and models deployed within the field and the increasing incorporation of explicit thinking about values into improvement research and practice.

The diversity of models and frameworks developed over this period (and briefly summarized in Section 1.2) springs in part from the changing social and cultural context of healthcare and – overlapping with that – the broadening disciplinary base of the field. There has also been a corresponding growth in practical expertise, drawing upon context-responsive 'informal reasoning'. Crudely speaking, the formalized methods and frameworks provide more-or-less sophisticated improvement 'recipes', but there is a clear understanding within the field – at least amongst experienced players – that there is a lot more to successful improvement work than following a recipe. While the emphasis on models or organizing frameworks makes the field sound ordered, rational and rule-following, these frameworks typically make space for context-sensitive adaptability and the 'soft skills' of relationship-building and dialogue. Discussions with improvers in broader practice contexts further emphasize this and it is worth noting that the methods that won 'silver' and 'bronze' in the 'Improvement Olympics' mentioned earlier (after PDSA cycles in first place) both place the values of collaboration and inclusion centre-stage. In practice improvement thinking is not confined to steadfastly technical mindsets but accommodates an interest in culture and values.

Attention to values and the value-laden nature of improvement is also, in some cases, reflected in the broadening of the field's disciplinary base. Whereas many of the original roots of improvement studies sit within a broadly technicist paradigm – heavily based upon lenses from psychology, management or other scientific-technical disciplines such as ergonomics – over time this paradigm has come to be qualified, challenged and complemented by other perspectives. Similarly, improvement methods now draw upon a more liberal range of feeder disciplines including design studies, sociology and social movement theory. Davina Allen and colleagues, for example, give an account of the growing contribution of sociology to healthcare improvement that acknowledges a body of sociological work that partially aligns with and strengthens the traditionally dominant technical paradigm but also celebrates the potentially disruptive potential generated by sociological voices that are interested in critical analysis as well as intervention.[25] They suggest that the historically dominant paradigm tended to treat healthcare 'quality' as a concrete thing that could be measured and managed in ways that fail to recognize the character of the social world. Understanding healthcare on an alternative, sociological paradigm means studying the political contexts of services, attending to power hierarchies and inequalities and seeing health systems as culturally differentiated and embodying competing values and interests. This means recognizing that the 'material' being shaped by improvement interventions is neither particularly consistent nor tractable, with the implication that improvers should be proportionately cautious in making claims about their approaches. It also includes recognizing the perspectives and values of the range of people within health systems. Sociology is not *either* practically useful *or* critically questioning but can be both.

Sociological contributions, along with critical voices from social movements or advocacy groups and so on, not only help elucidate and reframe the challenges of delivering better healthcare but also encourage debate about what counts as better healthcare. Such contributions are thus helpful precursors to, and in some respects overlap with, the kind of contribution that we are proposing for applied philosophy. Although, without wishing to draw a complete demarcation line, there are important differences of focus and emphasis between sociological and philosophical treatment of norms, the sociological emphasis is usually on either explaining or critiquing norms whereas the philosophical emphasis is both to seek to clarify norms (and associated concepts) and to ask about their relative justifiability and the bases on which they might be justified.

The maturation of healthcare improvement as a field has allowed for normative and ethical discussions to be brought into conversation with technical ones. Here it could either be said that the field has moved beyond assembling 'tools' or that it is now incorporating tools of critical analysis – tools that do a different kind of job but one that still has practical relevance.

1.5 Interrogating improvement

Against this background, this book asks some foundational philosophical questions about healthcare improvement. We have begun the work in this chapter by asking about the meaning and scope of healthcare improvement, and by highlighting different ways of thinking, and making judgements, about what counts as an improvement. When healthcare improvement is considered relatively narrowly, from a delivery perspective and within a technical paradigm, the assessment of improvement is largely translated into a set of empirical questions.[26] Studies are designed and executed to find out why those services that are deemed to work well do so. Similarly, the question of how to apply and spread relevant 'success conditions' can also be studied empirically and combined with 'know-how' drawn from leadership, management and other more applied, practice-facing fields. In a technical paradigm, questions about what counts as better and why, and especially the many uncertainties and possible disagreements about those questions, are not a central focus of study. Of course, questions about standards, norms or values are always somehow encompassed as one element of empirical work – by necessity some standards, norms or values must be assumed or specified, but they are largely defined in order to enable technical progress, rather than to facilitate ethical discussion or debate. Something like a technical paradigm is relatively suited to addressing delivery challenges. But the co-existence of revisionary questions, which challenge assumptions about what healthcare systems and actors ought to be doing, highlights the need to focus some attention on value questions and uncertainties alongside factual questions and uncertainties.

Ethical issues are important within both narrower and more expansive conceptions of healthcare improvement, but ethics will likely have contrasting framings and scope in each case. In relation to narrower conceptions, ethical issues might be construed in the same way that they often are characterized in biomedical contexts as a crucially important set of 'parallel concerns' that suggest some constraints on the implementation of an intervention. For example, as well as answering technical questions about the effectiveness of an intervention – 'Does fluoridation reduce dental decay?' – we need to decide whether or not the intervention is, or can be made, ethically acceptable – 'under what circumstances is fluoridation ethically permissible or required?' More expansive conceptions of improvement incorporate concern with the ethical acceptability of 'means' but also include interrogation of possible purposes, background values and judgement criteria, asking questions not just about the intervention or practice as given, but about underlying assumptions about what good practice entails. If we want to judge whether an intervention makes things better, we need to examine and analyse the (various competing) bases for this judgement (in combination with empirical questions about 'what happens when'). This moves ethics close to the centre of the field.

An important worry arises, however. Someone might well respond to this account by saying that a technical paradigm is designed first and foremost to be practical – to help decide upon and steer action. Talk of making space for analysis of value disagreements and uncertainties seems to threaten practical progress and so is seriously problematic. The concerned person might say that the ways of thinking needed to progress healthcare improvement are just different from those that belong in an ethics or philosophy seminar and are rightly kept separate. We take this possible reaction seriously and think there is something sound contained within it. We suggest, however, that the concern it expresses should be seen as something to navigate rather than a roadblock.

We accept that there can be a role sometimes for 'suspending' value discussion and for fixing, at least temporarily, the terms of reference used for planning and evaluating improvement practices. But this is not the same as denying the relevance of normative debate or analysis in the field. Indeed, this chapter has already indicated that in many respects healthcare improvement already operates from an expansive paradigm rather than a purely technical one. This is evident from the established contributions of sociologists, the growth of methods that engage with the values and perspectives of stakeholders and the broader incorporation of revisionary perspectives in the field. And improvement work sits within a public and policy context in which healthcare values and norms are, in any case, routinely called into question.

Our hope is to extend 'constructive scepticism' about healthcare improvement. In a sense the whole field of improvement is permeated with scepticism. It begins from questioning the way healthcare services are organized and enacted and by developing practical methods to improve them. The rise of sciences of improvement and accompanying scholarship reflects a further level of scepticism based on questioning the knowledge base of improvement practice and seeking to refine and extend it. Calls for a more scientific, 'objective' basis for claims about what good healthcare practice looks like can be interpreted as calls for rigour, peer review and critique. On the one hand, this involves highlighting the ways in which the subjective and perspectival experience of people working in healthcare can lead them to misguided ideas about good care. But, on the other hand, it also leads to questioning the adequacy of improvement and implementation methods. Do they, even collectively, provide a sufficiently rich framework for thinking about healthcare improvement? More concretely, when they are applied in practice are they, in specific cases, 'fit for purpose', sufficiently specified, applied with adequate fidelity and so on? The answer to the latter question will no doubt vary from case to case but there is a legitimate general risk that these models can serve to create an impression of tidy thinking when the underlying practices and service challenges are inherently complicated and messy.

Such concerns have been articulated within the improvement field. For example, the shortcomings of much current QI – some key grounds for scepticism – were illuminatingly summarized in 'Does quality improvement improve quality' by Mary Dixon-Woods and Graham Martin.[27] These include the frequency with which QI is thought about and enacted in short-term and small-scale ways – underpinned by an assumption that specific 'interventions' operate like 'magic bullets'. This tendency for the field to operate through multiple discrete projects with a heavy emphasis on innovation rather than replication – what Dixon-Woods and Martin call 'projectness' – reflects significant theoretical and strategic deficits. At a theoretical level, the underlying model fails to recognize the ways in which the effectiveness of QI initiatives – or of any action in a social field for that matter – needs to be seen as a product of the interactions between initiative and context, such that neat distinctions between the two, and especially hasty and tidy assumptions about causation, must be problematized. At a strategic level 'projectness' is a potential liability because it fails to consider how interventions may interact or have benefits at one level (e.g. within a unit) but cause problems at another (e.g. across an institution or system).

There are many other ways in which the improvement field is already questioning itself. Some critically reflexive improvers are asking, for example, what other institutional ends are served by talk of improvement? In the real world, institutions have many reasons to claim they are engaging in improvement – such as economic, political or public relations reasons – that can obscure what is going on within them. What are the unwanted or unanticipated effects of, or harms caused by, healthcare improvement (either by the way it is framed or by the way it is conducted)? Improvement activity itself uses financial and human resources and thus has 'costs' which cannot be neglected, including sometimes adding to the load and cumulative stress faced by people who in addition to trying to provide healthcare might also be under pressure to improve what is being done.[28] To the extent that people who are setting out to make healthcare better are not doing so and/or are in some ways having the reverse effect this is a matter of serious public and ethical concern.

We see the potential contribution of philosophy to healthcare improvement as promoting rigour by reinforcing, and expanding the scope of, these self-critical currents and tendencies. These existing currents mean that, in addition to the technical dimension in the field, there is also what might already be labelled in a general sense as a 'philosophical' dimension. Both dimensions are necessary to doing a good job. Our aims include: (a) to ensure that the existing 'philosophical dimension' is given due prominence on the map of the healthcare improvement field; (b) to more fully consider the interface between technical and philosophical dimensions of improvement; and (c) to make more explicit and open up some of the main philosophical and ethical questions facing the field, drawing more directly on the field of applied philosophy and ethics.

Healthcare improvement actors will often have a strong sense that they need to make improvements; by contrast, sceptical scholarly perspectives may suggest that such actors do not have a firm basis on which to act. One conclusion might be that a good deal of what goes on in the name of improvement should perhaps not take place. Another risk is that values and concerns that ought to be reflected in the mainstream of healthcare improvement are, in practice, relatively marginal. Being ready to embrace these radical conclusions is important. Those who work on improvements in health policy and services do not have the luxury of being able to step aside from thinking about these issues. Our hope is to show that thinking about improvement will be strengthened by more open and extensive engagement with conceptual and ethical issues, ideally with such engagement being seen as intrinsic to the field.

2 ACKNOWLEDGING COMPLEXITY

2.1 Does it work and is it a good idea?

Healthcare improvement as a practice typically involves identifying a way in which healthcare might be better, taking steps designed to bring that about, and monitoring or measuring to see how well these steps have worked. In this chapter we develop our account of the relationship between a more conventional empirical approach to the study of improvement and the more normatively conscious approach we propose in this book. Using an example of an improvement intervention and study, we show how any claim that some change amounts to an improvement is value-laden and open to contestation, being grounded in a series of assumptions about what matters and why. We explore what it means to say that an improvement process 'works' and whether, or on what interpretations, 'working' is a sufficient justification for taking further action, such as implementing new practices more permanently or widely. We suggest that behind technical assessments about whether an intervention 'works' are more holistic sets of assumptions or judgements about what counts as working and what is 'better'. These include assumptions and judgements about the scope of the system in question, its purposes and characteristics, and how these could evolve over time, as well as about the range of things that matter, why they matter (either instrumentally or for their own sake), how much they matter and from whose perspective such assessments should be made.

The chapter sets out some of the challenges involved in making healthcare improvement claims. It highlights two kinds of complexity that characterize claims about improvement: *explanatory* or causal complexity and *normative* complexity. We argue that these two kinds of complexity intersect and need to be considered together. While the importance of explanatory complexity is recognized in the field, normative complexity, and the added challenges it represents, deserves more attention. We use the language of 'explanatory complexity' as shorthand for the complexities attached to judging 'what causes what'. We use 'normative complexity' as shorthand for the complexities involved in judging that a change is an improvement – that is, that a service is better with or because of that change. Improvers can ask two related but distinct questions about any proposed improvement intervention: (a) does it work? – meaning something like 'does it do what it is intended to do?'; and (b) is it a good idea? – here meaning something like first, 'does it make things better?', and second, even assuming it does make things better in some respects, 'should we do it?'

2.2 The example – encouraging screening for social needs in primary healthcare

We begin by introducing our illustrative example. We have selected an example that is based on the premise that more might be done from within healthcare services to both recognize and address the social determinants of health (SDOH) – social conditions and experiences that directly or indirectly impact people's health. More specifically we look at an intervention designed to increase the extent to which primary care clinicians elicit and respond to their patients' housing and social isolation needs. We refer to this example, investigated and reported by Colleen Gillespie and colleagues, as 'the SDOH screening study'.[1] Although we are sympathetic to this kind of project, for the purpose of this chapter we are consciously neither endorsing nor critiquing it but rather exploring the ways that it illuminates both explanatory and normative complexity. We will first explore the difficulties attached to answering the 'does it work?' question. We will then look at what is involved in moving from 'does it work?' to 'is it a good idea?', and consider how these two questions connect.

We use the SDOH screening study as a springboard for raising concerns about evaluating healthcare improvement practice that could be applied to other scenarios, interventions and approaches. Clearly no single example can adequately represent the vast range of possibilities in healthcare improvement, and we do not pretend it does. We describe the study in some detail, but we are not fixed on the details of this or any particular case. For scientific purposes it would be crucial to represent all such details accurately but for our purposes we can, at times, afford to exercise some licence, and we make some imagined variations to slightly broaden its illustrative value.

The SDOH screening study asked how primary care doctors dealt with patients who presented health concerns and were also experiencing certain kinds of social need. It considered how much and how well doctors elicited, noticed and responded to social needs. And, specifically, it investigated whether providing audit-based feedback and some education increased the likelihood that doctors would both identify and meaningfully respond to these needs. The study authors report that the improvement intervention led to a statistically significant increase in screening, response and referral rates.

The SDOH screening study monitored practice both pre- and post-intervention. To audit doctors' practices, it used 'secret shopper' patients who were trained to present conditions and experiences in a standardized way. The patient actors each took on one of six 'presenting scenarios' that combined some overt medical concern (e.g. asthma exacerbation or shoulder pain) with both a housing and an isolation concern (e.g. mould or overcrowding and no friends or relationship breakdown). The relevant social concerns were not presented by the patient unless they were elicited by the doctor. The patient actors recorded if and how the social concerns were elicited and managed including through audiotape and an extensive checklist completed after each visit. The study took place in five primary care teams in one urban community with broadly comparable patient populations and where the use of patient actors was established. One of the five teams, selected at random, did not receive the intervention and served as a comparison group. The four teams in the intervention group received three audit reports, each including some education input, spaced over a nine-month period. The reports – in writing and presented verbally with an opportunity for discussion – were focused on teams rather than individual doctors. They first reported the measured screening and response rates, then introduced options for referral to social work and community services, provided guidance on the official documentation and data administration of SDOH categories, and followed up with information on the availability and positive value of referral options and other resources to help address social needs.

The monitoring of screening and referral rates showed changes in the intervention sites not matched in the comparison site. The rate of clinical staff eliciting housing need increased from less than half to 60 per cent, along with the exploration of and responses to the housing need rising from as little as 15 per cent to 41 per cent. There was a similar increase in the rate of eliciting social isolation but no equivalent rise in the rate of exploring and responding to that category of need. This improvement intervention was therefore largely successful at changing the behaviour of doctors and, furthermore, it is easy to see how this kind of study also indicates possible impacts of healthcare improvement. For example, it sheds light on the potential to strengthen the capabilities and knowledge of clinical staff, to better link together and 'coordinate' a range of services, and thereby to make care more responsive to patients.

We can imagine variations to the SDOH screening study in which one or more element is changed. For example, a different intervention could have been used (instead of audit-based feedback and education, perhaps a strengthening of local guidance linked to incentives); or the screening and referral being promoted could have been targeted at a specific kind of disease; or a very similar intervention could have taken place in a different healthcare setting such as in secondary care. The example arguably combines the two overlapping currents of improvement motivation introduced in Chapter 1. In some respects it sits clearly within what we have called a *delivery* conception of improvement, which typically involves deploying improvement interventions to increase the technical quality and consistency of clinical interventions. In contrast to many delivery-type improvement interventions, however, the SDOH screening study is not about closing the gap between a widely accepted standard and 'failing' services; rather, it is directed towards a somewhat *revisionary* conception of improvement utilizing a broader social interpretation of healthcare purposes than is commonplace. Even assuming the idea that primary care doctors should respond to social needs is quite widely accepted in principle, it is well short of an accepted expectation in practice.[2]

2.3 Scepticism and uncertainty about improvement claims and interventions

The SDOH screening study authors go to some lengths to establish that the improvement intervention worked. It is not easy to justify a claim of this sort and, for it to be made with reasonable confidence, such a claim must be a suitably specific and defined one. The authors claim that the intervention is capable of modifying certain healthcare activities, such as the tendency for doctors to discuss social needs with their patients. They do not claim that these changes to healthcare practice will necessarily lead in turn to specific desired outcomes, such as people's social needs being met. The latter is quite a different claim and, obviously, a much more ambitious one. However, the significance of the intervention is that it rests on the idea that the practice change would increase the likelihood of the health and care system addressing people's social needs and so anyone making claims about it succeeding as an improvement intervention must give some attention to that broader canvas.

Making the claim that a healthcare improvement intervention 'works' usually depends upon the use of social science research methods (in combination with clinical and/or public health sciences). These, in turn, depend upon ontological, epistemological and methodological assumptions and commitments – that is, assumptions and commitments about what there is, what people can know and how they can come to know it.[3] In general terms, an improvement researcher claiming that 'x improvement intervention has worked' faces the same kind of demands as a pharmaceutical researcher claiming that 'x drug or device has worked', although there are specific challenges – both ethical and epistemological – to producing such claims in predominantly social rather than physical or biological arenas. Roughly speaking these challenges stem from the ways that it is difficult to extend anything even analogous to 'laboratory conditions' into the social world of healthcare improvement. Here we will briefly note the ethical challenges and say a little more about the epistemic challenges which are central to the theme of this chapter.

The SDOH screening study adopts a quasi-experimental design and there are limits to how far it is ethically acceptable to conduct 'social experiments' on people outside of contexts like clinical trials where there are embedded safeguards such as consent procedures. The epistemic challenges arise because social reality is highly variegated. Social worlds vary across space and time and continuously evolve culturally and structurally. Both the immediate and the broader contexts in which interventions take place are thus diverse and in flux. The SDOH example is arguably 'doubly difficult' in this regard. If the screening triggered a pharmaceutical or therapeutic intervention with a very strong evidence-base, this element of the picture would seem somewhat less socially contingent and less distant from laboratory science. This would be closer to an ideal starting point in implementation sciences – one in which there is good evidence for a clinical intervention and the challenge is to research and identify a good combination of strategies for achieving its uptake. Within improvement research there is increasing recognition of the need to think about interventions taking place in complex and 'open' social systems that make it difficult to make predictions about effects or even to identify potential causal pathways that are clear or stable.[4] A complex, as opposed to complicated, system is typically characterized by many different interrelated components and a high number of unknowns, which make it difficult to control and predict and mean that it is not possible to reduce the system to codified rules and processes.[5] The design used in the SDOH screening study is one of a range of 'quasi-scientific' means of attenuating such 'explanatory complexity' by strongly circumscribing the system under investigation and limiting the range of factors under consideration.

Whilst fully recognizing the strengths and promise of this sort of improvement intervention it is also possible to raise sceptical questions about it, and these questions have wider relevance to improvement approaches. As already indicated in Section 2.1, we have in mind two broad and overlapping sets of questions. First, when are improvers justified in making claims that an intervention 'works' such that they can reasonably make causal claims about it and expect that it can be applied with something like the intended effects outside of the confines of a particular study and set of circumstances? Second, even when it seems clear that an intervention can have the results it is intended to have, what (else) is involved in deciding that it is a good idea and *should* be applied? Before deciding to recommend any kind of intervention to increase the rate of any kind of healthcare activity improvers would, at minimum, need provisional answers to these two sets of questions. The theme of the first set of questions is very familiar in the field of healthcare improvement and the applied social sciences more broadly. It often comes up in discussions within research methodology about the problem of 'generalizing' from specific studies (or 'external validity') and in relation to the ambition of 'scaling up' or 'spreading' interventions that have been successful in one set of circumstances but seem to warrant more general application. The theme of the second set of questions is much less prominent in the healthcare improvement literature (which is the reason we concentrate on it here). However, as we go on to discuss in the next section, answers to these two sets of questions are entangled in ways that make it difficult and unhelpful to try to fully separate them out.

In making and attempting to justify claims about improvement, improvers will likely have in mind that the healthcare activity itself works and serves at least one valuable end, and that the improvement intervention works to increase the rate or quality of the activity such that the improvement intervention increases the realization of valuable end(s). In other words, the basic reasoning here will often be something like A (an improvement intervention) is valuable because it leads to B (increased/improved healthcare activity) and B brings about or amounts to C (something of value). One critical complication that might arise for healthcare improvement – which we pass over relatively quickly at this point – is whether A (and/or B) might also be judged to have 'bad effects' (to be in some respects undesirable, harmful or even perhaps wrong), which must be balanced against the value of C. No interventions are 'cost-free'. They all use resources such as money, time and attention that might be used in other ways – sometimes labelled the 'opportunity cost' of an intervention – so judging that C will be achieved is never, on its own, sufficient for recommending A. There is always some element of having to balance competing considerations together. In the second half of this chapter, and especially in the rest of the book, we explore more fully what 'balancing competing considerations' can entail. For now, it is enough to note that it includes managing potential tensions between: (a) different, and sometimes competing, ends including (b) shorter and longer-term ends, and (c) more narrowly defined and more broadly conceived ends.

Evaluating a specific improvement intervention thus gives rise to intersecting clusters of uncertainty. These might be crudely classified as (1) empirical and (2) 'value' uncertainties (although, as we discuss later, this is not a tidy separation):

1   Does A lead to B, and B to C? With what certainty? What other
    'side effects' arise from A and B?

2   Is C valuable and, if so, how valuable and why? How undesirable
    or desirable are the other features and effects of A and B, and
    why?

Making judgements about the effects and value of interventions
is challenging. We have already introduced some of the difficulties
of tracing patterns of causation in complex social systems. There are
analogous difficulties attached to determining what is valuable. There
is widespread disagreement about what matters, and what matters
more, in evaluating healthcare. Actions can be valued (favourably
or unfavourably) for what they embody or represent independently
of their causal effects, and such valuations can vary according to an
individual's standpoint. We will come back to this idea briefly later
in this chapter (and discuss it more fully in later chapters) but one
example is whether health professionals treat people respectfully (or
disrespectfully) – something people attach value to independently of
the (varied) consequences it might produce. Making practical evaluative
judgements often involves trading off or balancing different values which
cannot practically co-exist or be pursued simultaneously, as well as
managing both 'empirical' and 'value' uncertainties. And the way these
two kinds of uncertainties are handled are related. If improvers judge
that the desired effects of an intervention are only marginally valuable,
they are probably going to need quite a high threshold of confidence
that planned improvement activities will bring them about and that the
activities are relatively low cost or raise few negative concerns. To the
extent that improvers feel seriously uncertain about the combinations
of effects that an intervention might bring about, they are going to be in
a difficult position to assess its value.

From the account we have given of the SDOH screening study, it is
not clear how likely it is that the improvement intervention will have its
desired effects, nor exactly what kinds of effects these are and in what
sense they are valuable. In the next section we explore one key factor in
assessing improvement claims: the scope and context of judgements of
improvement. That is, how narrow or wide should the frame of reference
be set when judging whether an intervention works and whether it is a
good idea? Any answer will involve empirical claims about the range of
valued effects that an improvement intervention might generate, but it

will also likely require some consideration of how to characterize some of the 'valued ends' at stake. This latter set of issues will gradually become our focus in the rest of the chapter.

2.4 Judging improvement in context

The audit and educational feedback intervention in the SDOH screening study can reasonably be viewed as being informed by, and making a contribution to, a broader vision of how healthcare services might be improved. The chance of this improvement intervention being successful in the broader sense of addressing SDOH and contributing to the health and well-being of patients depends on there being effective social, community and housing services or equivalent voluntary support agencies that can pick up and build effectively on the screening practices, referrals and responses of the primary care teams. Without this condition being met, the improvement intervention might work in a narrow technically defined sense but largely fail to work in a more expansive and meaningful sense. Indeed, if the health professionals whose practices are targeted for improvement are sceptical about the broader enabling conditions being in place, they may well anticipate this obstacle and, especially over time, may screen and refer less, thereby undercutting the improvement intervention's success even in the narrowest sense. Even if the relevant conditions were in place in the context of the study, other contexts might well be different – perhaps having much less extensive and effective services or substantially different configurations of services that produce different (not necessarily worse but different) sets of outcomes.

It is a well-established principle in the evaluation of all screening policies that unless there are suitable services in place to deal effectively with referrals, an introduction of screening or increase in screening rates will not amount to much of an improvement, even if the screening is 'effective' in the narrowly defined sense of identifying problems.[6] Indeed, where referrals cannot be dealt with, providing screening is arguably a *disservice* because it raises expectations which the system fails to meet – guiding people down a false path. For example, it could be argued that the threat of a 'screening disservice' might apply to the SDOH screening study in relation to social isolation needs where detection rates increased but referral rates did not. This is one potential criticism of at least this aspect of the screening intervention, that is, it encouraged social isolation screening when perhaps it should not have done so. The authors downplay the clinicians' lack of response, but also risk accepting the validity of the 'disservice' criticism by explaining that 'there is, currently, a lack of consensus on and insufficient evidence for how best to intervene in addressing loneliness and social isolation'.[7] This raises the question of when it is defensible to encourage screening despite a lack of agreement or policy about what follows the screening.

It might, however, be argued that improvers should be judging the potential contribution of interventions in an even broader context – thinking not only about what existing patterns of services happen to be like, but about what they could and should be, or at least what seems feasible given planned policy change. Service improvements can be conceived and judged not only on knowledge about existing system configurations but also on the basis of assumptions about the trajectories of systems and services. It is not a serious criticism of someone constructing a railway line to say that the track stops just two miles after it starts if the reasonable expectation is that others will soon be constructing another part of the line that meets it there. There are, however, usually very substantial uncertainties about the nature and success of planned and future activities, especially in often volatile policy domains such as public transport or healthcare.

This provides the basis for a possible response to the 'screening disservice' concern. The SDOH screening study examines the extent to which clinicians in one setting currently do, and potentially could, recognize and respond to social needs. Given concerted and collaborative efforts for health and care systems to address social needs, including social isolation – by, for example, better connecting healthcare settings with communities and community services – it is possible that more meaningful and widespread responses to social isolation may be put in place (e.g. perhaps through forms of 'social prescribing') to complement and warrant the increased emphasis on screening for isolation. In other words, change has to start somewhere, and this specific study might be seen as one piece of a bigger whole – as sitting within a broader policy movement that is aimed at reconfiguring or rebalancing the orientation of health services.

Judgements about what might count as 'working' can alter as the frame of reference is opened up in the way we have illustrated. However, expanding the frame of reference highlights two significant complications. First, it underlines the relatively limited value of the findings of this kind of study to drawing conclusions about the real-world contribution of an intervention. That is, in order to determine whether this screening intervention could have broader benefits than 'merely' changing the activities of doctors in comparable circumstances, improvers need to know, or make assumptions, about many other things. Second, the assumptions improvers need to make or the knowledge they need to have – for example, about service trajectories and policy directions – relate not only to what is feasible but also to what is desirable. Most obviously this includes assumptions or knowledge about whether and how health services should address social needs. Closely circumscribing the focus of a study to partly bypass explanatory complexity and to yield reliable answers to some carefully specified questions comes at the price of 'bracketing out' normative as well as explanatory complexity if assumptions about what matters are not explicitly deliberated or identified.

'Zooming out' from the details of a particular example and thinking about the wider system and policy context bring normative questions and uncertainties into view. Someone who was being conscientiously sceptical might raise many doubts about the example intervention or other comparable interventions. Should clinicians be encouraged to screen for social needs? Should it be part of their role? Do they have the appropriate expertise, and sufficient time and resources, to do it well? Might there be other settings and kinds of roles where this might be done better? If there was action elsewhere could this reduce the need for screening and referrals? Even if improvers agree that screening in primary care settings makes good sense, they could still ask: (a) How far should this assumption be applied to clinicians in other settings (should it always be part of the role of doctors, and if not, when should it be included/excluded)? (b) Should it be relatively prioritized in the training of clinicians, or service reform, or are there other improvements that should take priority? Such questions suggest ways in which the ostensive value of improvement interventions, when seen through a narrow frame, can merit additional investigation or require further justification when wider frames are brought into consideration.

To illustrate further, imagine two contrasting sceptics – Amy and Zack. Amy thinks that primary care screening for social needs is an excellent idea in principle but that in her location the community services and support needed to make it successful in practice are simply not in place. In her setting, Amy thinks that the kind of primary care intervention we are discussing is not just a waste of resource but would add to the frustrations of people struggling with inadequate housing and social isolation and is, therefore, the wrong thing to do. Zack feels that there might be a place for such screening under some circumstances but that the first priority should be neither health-sector-based screening nor community welfare services but much more investment in the social fabric and infrastructure including housing, alongside redistributive welfare policies. Zack thinks advocates for meeting social needs should be wary of the risk of 'medicalizing' social needs by resorting too quickly to clinically prescribed 'sticking plasters'. From both perspectives it could be argued that interventions to promote certain forms of screening are undesirable – either simply because they waste resources and create false expectations, or because they obscure better, perhaps more radical, measures that ought to be taken elsewhere by other agencies or actors.

The imagined positions of Amy and Zack are far removed from the carefully specified technical framing of the SDOH case study. In a technically framed account, both the conceptualization of the improvement intervention and the criteria of success applied to it are tightly defined. This level of specification supports improvers in making relatively confident claims about an intervention working (drawing on some appropriate conventions of research rigour). If, however, improvers are interested in the broader practical question of whether a possible healthcare improvement intervention should be pursued (whether it is a 'good idea') then things become very much more complicated.

2.5 What makes an improvement intervention a good idea?

We now turn explicitly to the broader question of when an improvement intervention ought to be pursued. Drawing on the SDOH screening study we have already indicated that the screening is motivated by some presumed health system goal(s) ('C') and noted that some people may question the desirability of the improvement intervention ('A') and its immediate effect of increasing rates of screening for social need ('B'). Here we will focus in more closely both on the issue of how, why and whether C is valuable as well as some of the factors that might have to be balanced against that. Asking these questions about identifying and valuing purposes, and balancing different considerations together, highlights the existence of multiple competing conceptions of 'good healthcare', and therefore of what counts as improving healthcare.

One way to approach these questions might be to ask in general terms about the purposes of healthcare, including how far prevention, rather than treatment, or the addressing of social need rather than clinical or biomedical need, should be the role of healthcare services. This might also include related analyses of definitions of health and in what respects health can be clearly distinguished from well-being. This is one potentially helpful means of bringing a philosophical lens into this area (and is explored in Chapter 8). While some progress can be made like this, it would likely be insufficient to resolve the normative uncertainties in the example we are discussing. For example, in clarifying the possible aims of healthcare useful conceptual distinctions could be made between prevention and treatment, health and well-being, and so on but (a) there would be ongoing disagreements about how best to make such distinctions, (b) there is no reason to suppose such distinctions would map neatly onto the roles of health service workers because institutions and roles need to be organized partly around pragmatic rather than conceptual distinctions and (c) answering questions about aims or purposes does not neatly precede engagement with empirical questions about feasibility or the specific historical circumstances and affordances of actual health systems. To some extent, questions about what services ought to aim for and do are contingent on what it is realistically possible for them to do. In short, we have reservations about pursuing 'foundational' philosophical questions in abstraction from empirical questions. These are somewhat analogous to reservations others might have about pursuing practical-ethical questions about improvement without first addressing more foundational questions about key healthcare concepts and values. We are suggesting that improvers need to engage explicitly with conceptual and ethical questions and that they need to so in relation to particular cases and contexts (not only in the abstract) and whilst accepting that such questions will remain to some degree contentious.

What could make the kind of improvement envisaged in the SDOH screening study valuable? Improvers could narrow the field of answers (for now) by assuming that the important answers are not to do with the effects of the improvement intervention on the capabilities and practices of primary care teams but on potential benefit to the lives and well-being of patients. But focusing in more detail on what might make SDOH screening valuable indicates that there is no simple answer. Both narrower clinical and broader social ends might be served and there is nothing like a clear separation between them; rather, the clinical and social are intertwined. And, furthermore, there are multiple kinds of ways in which referrals and responses to SDOH needs could be valuable – including being instrumentally valuable in relation to other valued ends, but also being valuable in their own right.

Although it is not expressed in these terms, the complex value of SDOH screening becomes quickly evident on reading the study report. The scenarios presented by the actor-patients are designed to combine some overt health-related symptoms or conditions with social needs and the working assumption is that the latter – as the SDOH label makes explicit – are equally relevant to health. The introduction of the paper provides a useful overview indication and some illustrations of this relevance:

> [C]onnecting a patient with food insecurity to a meal programme can enable them to focus on adhering to medication or attend follow-up appointments rather than on their more immediate need for food. Helping a patient obtain more secure or better quality housing can decrease exposure to associated health risks (eg, toxic conditions, violence, substance use, infectious disease), decrease stress overall and therefore directly enhance health, and/or provide patients with the stability to more effectively manage their health. Social isolation may exacerbate existing depression or result from untreated depression. Care can also be adjusted to compensate for social needs (social risk-informed care), for example, by sending a patient who has problems with transportation their prescription by mail and thereby minimising the deleterious impact of that social need. Failure to acknowledge and/or address these social needs increases care costs, can compromise patient safety and is oftentimes viewed as an indicator of poor quality healthcare … Without identification, such needs cannot be adequately addressed in clinical care, leading to the risk of ineffective treatment (e.g., prescribing medications the patient can't pay for, recommending behaviour changes the patient's environment doesn't support, failing to incorporate air quality into the assessment of a patient's report of breathing problems).[8]

This passage helpfully illuminates some of the ways in which those working in healthcare settings can, and indeed it seems ought to, be mindful of broader social environments as well as the social constraints patients face. Simplistically, SDOH screening is instrumentally valuable because it brings about improved health. But the quoted passage helpfully indicates the diverse ways in which this might manifest in practice: preventing health risks and exacerbation of health conditions, protecting patient safety, enhancing health services accessibility and responsiveness, enabling better (more informed) diagnoses and more effective treatment and disease management (through, for example, more appropriate prescribing or better supported self-management) and reducing demands on patients which prevent them from attending to their health needs. This indicative list highlights part of the challenge of answering the 'is it a good idea?' question about SDOH-related interventions. There are many potentially valuable things at stake, and it is often unclear which are seen, and should be seen, as most valuable; which combinations of them are being sought; and whether all or any of them might be achievable in practice.

The purposes summarized in the extracted passage above are formulated in ways that reflect typical health service agendas. They are, in short, either about better health outcomes or better-run health services. For work targeted at healthcare and health professionals this is understandable. It may also partly reflect service user perspectives and needs, at least as far as their health is concerned. But, on further reflection, there is something missing from this account. It might be thought that an interest in addressing social needs can be justified without reference to health at all. The idea of a social need points to something that requires addressing for people to be enabled to live their lives with a decent level of well-being.[9] In the case of housing or social isolation needs, as deployed in the example, people's well-being is clearly undermined by having to live in damp or overcrowded conditions or by having very few social contacts and experiencing loneliness even if this is not causing them to be unhealthy in ways that are conventionally clinical or health service concerns. Steps that might be taken to acknowledge and address these needs seem to be valuable for their own sake and for the sake of people's well-being, and not simply because of their important potential health benefits.

The expected and desired benefits of SDOH screening are only part of the picture. There are also various risks and costs to bear in mind. Leaving aside economic cost–benefit considerations for now, we have, for example, already touched upon worries about creating false expectations and the medicalization of social need. Some researchers have published quite hard-hitting critiques of clinical screening for social need that include and extend these worries. For example, Arvin Garg and colleagues warn of the dangers of such screening reinforcing aspects of health inequality and potentially producing experiences of discrimination, stigma and feelings of shame.[10] These, they argue, can be products of incorporating a focus on poverty into powerful clinical institutions and roles unless the measures introduced with such a focus are developed in partnership with relevant communities, according to carefully considered standards and enacted by health professionals with both empathy and humility. Their argument amounts to saying that a 'revisionary' approach that incorporates social needs in clinical spaces needs to be accompanied by a revision of norms that displaces the centrality of clinical categories and power or at least extends such categories so that they are based on greater mutuality and equality between service providers and service users. The upshot is that making judgements about what is valuable in this kind of case depends both upon *how* interventions are introduced and how far improvers are prepared to revisit their evaluative lenses. All of this underlines the contestability of claims about what is valuable. It is far from obvious how improvers should 'think across' (reason about, combine, choose between or balance) the diverse range of things that matter when designing or evaluating improvement interventions. There are many possibilities for doing so, given that improvement activities can proceed, implicitly or explicitly, with various contrasting conceptions of what counts as good healthcare.

Up to now we have been assuming that the value of encouraging clinicians to screen for and respond to social needs is instrumental: it leads to improved health, well-being, material welfare or other valued ends. It is at least worth noting that clinicians showing an interest in, exploring and making suggestions about patients' experiences of poor housing or social isolation could also be valuable in itself. This is arguably something of central importance for understanding and evaluating health services. Healthcare is not simply about technical interventions but also about 'care' and relationships, and at least part of the value of relationships – what they express, the goods they embody, the way they 'feel' – is independent of any health outcomes that follow from interventions.[11] It might be better for a clinician not only to meaningfully engage with and take seriously a person's experience of isolation but also to be able to do something that helps 'fix' it. But acknowledging people's social needs and taking them seriously may also be valuable because it expresses respect and recognition for them in important ways – and perhaps especially so for someone who feels isolated and 'unheard'. This is one respect in which a need can be responded to – albeit only partially and temporarily – for its own sake and not necessarily for health-related benefit. Assuming screening is done sensitively and sincerely and not as a 'tick box' exercise, this is another possible response to charges that screening that is not followed up by services lacks value. There might also be an analogous argument that the intervention used in the SDOH screening study – audit-based feedback plus education – could itself be of value irrespective of whether, as it happens, benefits flow to patients if it contributes significantly to the education, reflective practice and understanding of clinicians – something which is worthwhile for a variety of reasons not all of which relate to measurable patient benefit. These ways of looking beyond health outcome framings add to the difficulty of judging whether something is valuable and can be defended as a good idea.

Acknowledging the explanatory and normative complexities in this kind of case does not mean that it is impossible to come to any practical conclusions. For example, it seems perfectly reasonable to conclude that, on balance, there are good reasons to encourage suitably placed doctors to engage in screening for social needs, assuming it is done in ways that are empathic and do not undermine patients' dignity or psychological safety. Likewise, it may be valuable for clinicians to strengthen their links with other agencies that they can refer patients to and form partnerships with. Nonetheless, when considering whether a particular intervention is a good idea and ought to be encouraged, it seems better to think of any resulting claim as the conclusion of an argument or the endpoint of deliberation or reflection, rather than simply as an empirical discovery (where the latter might apply to a narrow interpretation of whether something has 'worked'). This way of thinking also has practical advantages because it reinforces the importance of proper discussion and critical reflection before improvers institute an intervention; and it means that, if they proceed, they will be sensitized to, and can be mindful about, recognized complications and counterarguments.

2.6 Opening up improvement concepts and ethics

We have begun to illustrate why conceptual and ethical issues are at the heart of healthcare improvement and have significant implications for researching and practising improvement. It is worth more explicitly underlining what we are saying. It is not merely that 'external' philosophical perspectives and voices could be 'added in' to the discourses and practices of healthcare improvement to provide additional intellectual resources for thinking about, planning or critiquing improvement efforts. Rather, practically important conceptual and ethical issues and positions are already and necessarily 'built into' the business of improvement. The choice improvers face is not about whether to embrace an extra 'feeder discipline' but whether to notice (or turn away from) this reality.

We have used the case study to draw out some of the contrasts between a broadly 'technicist' emphasis, which is commonplace in an empirical sciences approach to improvement, and a normatively conscious approach, which opens up more indeterminate questions and ways of thinking. These contrasts apply both to the way improvement agendas and aims are characterized and to the ways judgements are made about how, where and when to act. They apply, that is, both to the concepts improvers deploy and to the ethics of improvement practice. These two areas of emphasis are, respectively, the subjects of Parts 2 and 3 of the book. To conclude this chapter, we link our present discussion to each of these and introduce their significance.

Attention to the concepts deployed by improvers is important because fundamental normative questions and assumptions arise before even considering which interventions might be justified. As we have illustrated, healthcare services operate in social and policy contexts in which there are a range of potentially relevant purposes along with different readings of what is or can be valuable about healthcare processes. In short, there are ambiguities and contests about what counts as 'good healthcare' and, therefore, about what counts as better or worse. In the three chapters of Part 2, we will argue that the idea of 'quality' is inherently plural and that a serious engagement with healthcare improvement has to find ways of understanding and managing this pluralism. Acknowledging this is not just relevant at the level of an individual service – where there can be legitimate disagreement about the ways or extent to which the service is improving – but to system-wide coordination and coherence. There may be good reasons for different services to operate with different accounts of what is good, or constructions of healthcare quality, given, for example, that services can be oriented to different populations with different needs (social and clinical), may have different core aims (e.g. cure, rehabilitation, prevention) and may have historically 'fallen short' in diverse respects, some of which might also seem more quantifiable than others. In other words, pluralism is not merely a philosophically interesting question but also a practical ethical challenge for the evaluation and coordination of services.

If, for the sake of discussion, 'healthcare improvement' is taken to be shorthand for bringing about better healthcare and 'healthcare quality' is taken to be shorthand for good healthcare, then it is clear that these shorthand concepts are not easily defined and are heavily value-laden and contestable. Much of the discussion in this chapter, for example, has been about possible uncertainties and contests about the interpretation of 'effectiveness' in screening for social needs, and effectiveness is typically seen as a core (perhaps the core) dimension of healthcare quality. Within a carefully defined research framework improvers can specify what they mean by effectiveness ('what works', narrowly understood) but that kind of closure is not possible outside of an artificially framed conception of effectiveness, such as when reflecting on the success of health services more generally. Contests of this kind are multiplied when the range of normative complexity is brought into view, for example via: (a) similar debates about other aspects or dimensions of quality such as safety or equity; (b) questions about how to relatively prioritize and balance the range of valued quality dimensions; (c) the different impacts (including costs and benefits) that proposed changes may have on diverse sub-populations or groups; and (d) the way that different stakeholders (e.g. health service managers, professional groups, patient advocacy groups) might differently interpret and weight both these differential impacts and the different aspects of 'quality' or 'better care'.

It is easy to be misled by the fact that words like 'improvement' or 'quality' sound both singular and simple. Especially in a context where measurement is important it can easily seem that saying 'the quality of this service has been improved' is a bit like saying 'the height of this building has been increased'. But in real-world settings this equivalence will virtually never hold. It is, of course, possible – indeed almost inevitable – that any improvement intervention will make things better in some respects and from some perspectives but, at the same time, risks making things worse in some other respects and/or from other perspectives.

Someone hearing the phrase 'ethics of healthcare improvement' might well, and in many ways quite reasonably, imagine it refers to some specific subset of concerns. For example, they might frame it in the way that (institutionalized) research ethics is often framed: as highlighting a particular bundle of considerations (about informed consent, confidentiality, etc.) that must be addressed before and alongside conducting research. Or, overlapping with that, they might frame it as about conspicuously problematic or contentious questions that can arise in any activity – such as questions about the use of unacceptable procedures or the threat of harmful effects. In the SDOH screening study, for instance, ethical questions might arise about the use of 'secret shoppers' – did the clinicians fully understand and unequivocally agree to this? What would such agreement involve and how feasible is it? Similar ethical questions could also arise about the intervention, most obviously if it strayed from offering feedback and education. Would financial or other forms of incentives be acceptable, and if so, then what about using pay cuts as a disincentive? These are all ethical questions and are worthy of careful attention but they by no means indicate the full interface between improvement and ethics. Indeed, these framings suggest that ethical issues could, for the most part, be kept outside of improvement thinking. That is, they suggest that there might be a substantial space of practical reasoning about improvement that can fully proceed without any risk of getting 'bogged down' in addressing uncertainties about values and ethics. On this picture ethical thinking is relevant at the 'fringes' – either as a parallel concern that needs addressing to ensure improvement activities are authorized as socially acceptable and/or because some clearly contentious concern or dilemma comes into view.

By contrast our suggestion, developed in Part 3, is that there is no practical reasoning space which is not at the same time an ethical reasoning space. It is possible, and it may sometimes be helpful, to deliberately 'bracket out' normative questions for specific purposes but that is, in effect, an artificial exercise. In conceiving, planning and executing an improvement intervention, improvers are inevitably using value-laden concepts and, consciously or not, committing to one set of values rather than another set. It is accepted in healthcare improvement that improvers have to be accountable for their reasoning. They must, for example, be able to justify the basis on which they are claiming that something 'works'. Given an assumption of accountability, improvers might also reasonably be asked to account for how they have arrived (or could arrive) at the relevant value set. To this end, they would need to explain how and why they decided that *this* is what counts as an improvement and that *this* intervention, rather than none or something else, is a good idea. Their choice of both concepts and practices necessitates ethical thinking (which, for now, we roughly equate with 'deliberating about values'). Some value choices may be about fairly subtle discriminations but many of them are not – they concern what the core purposes of healthcare are, and hence what kinds of things are relative priorities.

In the SDOH screening study, for example, Gillespie and colleagues' assumption that it is the role of primary health services to screen for and respond to social needs embodies an ethical stance – a stance that can, of course, be questioned. Similarly, both the way that potential contribution is characterized, and the measures of success adopted, raise ethical questions. If clinicians ought to screen for social needs, is this because it can contribute to 'health outcomes', community well-being more generally, reductions in societal inequalities and/or to better practising of patient-centred consultations or experiences of being cared about? As we have noted each of these valued ends will significantly shape both the causal links improvers need to study and the ways they would evaluate success. Likewise, the form of intervention adopted, whilst relatively uncontroversial, is far from immune to ethical interrogation. It may be that improvers can find satisfactory answers to these questions about concepts and practices, but once they stand back from a narrow technical framing of interventions, they will confront normative complexity and uncertainty.

In this chapter, we have begun to indicate that judging whether something amounts to an improvement is not descriptively, causally or ethically straightforward. Even in the case of a very promising example, it is possible to raise doubts both about the extent to which something might form a successful intervention and about the various respects it can be said to make things better or worse. More generally we have started to explore the gap between evaluating improvement using a primarily scientific-technical lens and a more open-ended ethical lens. The former translates or 'operationalizes' improvement into measurable categories which enables a degree of clarity and confidence about the evaluation of success. The latter highlights the extent to which this operationalization involves normative and contestable judgements. We do not see these perspectives as alternatives; rather, they can be used in complementary ways.

The overlap between the scientific-technical and ethical perspectives connects to the limits of the fact-value distinction briefly mentioned in Chapter 1. Improvers can perfectly well talk about identifying relevant 'facts' through, for example, empirical research processes. But such facts will not somehow be 'shorn' of values. Even if such a thing is possible in some areas of inquiry (e.g. in characterizations of sub-atomic processes in physics) it certainly does not apply to descriptions of healthcare and social life which are saturated with values. To describe certain approaches as 'technicist' is to indicate that they proceed by attempting to artificially insulate empirical and value discriminations for practical purposes *as if that were possible*. Technical accounts may not appear explicitly value-laden or normative, but they will exhibit what has been called 'implicit normativity'[12] – a phenomenon we will discuss further in the following chapters. We have illustrated in this chapter that lying in the background of technical judgements about whether an intervention 'works' are more holistic sets of assumptions or judgements about what counts as working, including: (a) about the characteristics of the system one is working in and how these could evolve and (b) about what range of things matter and how much, either instrumentally or for their own sake, and as seen from different vantage points.

The SDOH screening study we have used as an example, including the use of a quasi-experiment, might be seen to exaggerate the contrast between empirical and normative frames of reference. There are many less 'technicist' approaches to empirical research, including within healthcare improvement. These include, for example, those that use qualitative methods or mixed and multiple methods, and that draw on and develop interdisciplinary theories of various kinds. There are also many approaches to improvement that recognize and respond to the variegated nature of the social world – sometimes by closely combining research and practice activities in ways that embrace the need for context-responsive adaptation including different styles of facilitation to help make interventions 'work' in different settings.[13] These approaches, as noted above, recognize the need to address explanatory complexity but they do not acknowledge, let alone address, normative complexity. If we had used an example of improvement research with less technicist characteristics we would have produced a slightly different story, but the same points would still be relevant. Empirical research that involves interpretive elements and/or which involves integrating elements from diverse kinds of data analysis and theoretical readings must more-or-less consciously address and manage the conceptual and ethical complications that we have rehearsed. If anything, what we have suggested about philosophical issues being 'built into' improvement research and practice is likely to be more evident when unpacking these other examples. Furthermore, having noted the more expansive and self-reflective tendencies in some forms of empirical research, there is always a risk that when research is 'translated' into practice, especially in contexts where biomedical conceptions of research are influential, many of these nuances are lost, such that 'findings' are still treated in essentially technicist ways (e.g. in formulations such as 'research shows that x works'). The contrast we have drawn between 'scientific-technical' conceptions of knowledge and more 'expansive' conceptions can apply to both research and practice, and it is not uncommon for research to align with broader interdisciplinary models but for a scientific-technical mindset to reassert itself as knowledge is utilized in practice.

The rather loose heuristic distinction that we have made between technical and ethical lenses on improvement has some resonances with the distinction introduced in Chapter 1 between 'delivery' and 'revisionary' improvement motivations. They are, however, separate distinctions and they intersect rather than coincide. Strengthening existing services and models of care, on the one hand, or rethinking and reorienting services and models, on the other, can be viewed through both technical and ethical lenses. One of the differences is that 'revisionary' agendas will typically arise from conscious exploration and debate about healthcare values and 'delivery' agendas may well not. Nonetheless they are equally based on value assumptions. In both cases using a technical lens can be helpful but, unless it is done with an awareness of the much less clear-cut interpretations, assumptions and contestations that sit in the background it can also be misleading.

In short, making judgements about putative improvements is complex. The existence of explanatory complexity – the difficulty of tracing what might lead to what combinations of effects – is well-recognized and the focus of significant epistemological and methodological attention. But, for those trying to decide what to do in practice, this form of complexity is overlaid and entangled with normative complexity – the challenges of determining what kinds of changes are 'improvements' and, more broadly, what is valuable in healthcare. Trying to acknowledge and address explanatory complexity is thus only part of what is needed. Indeed, improvers will not be in a position to make much progress with relevant empirical research unless they are at the same time ready to consider and discuss the range of things that matter, why they might matter, and how they consist of, or give rise to, competing concerns and values. Without such normative consciousness, they are much more likely to make mistakes in designing and directing empirical research, and in deciding what kinds of approaches and frames to deploy.

PART TWO

ANALYSING CONCEPTS

3 QUALITY IS PLURAL

The idea of 'quality' is commonly invoked in contemporary health policy, research and practice across the anglophone world, particularly when claims are being made about how good or bad healthcare services are, how well organizations or teams are performing and what kinds of improvement have been achieved or are needed. In England, the Care Quality Commission (CQC) is the independent regulator of health and social care, which has the responsibility of monitoring, inspecting and rating healthcare services; in Australia, the National Safety and Quality Health Service Standards provide a 'nationally consistent statement of the level of care consumers can expect from health service organizations'; in the United States the Agency for Healthcare Research and Quality is a Federal agency responsible for 'improving the safety and quality of healthcare for all Americans'.[1] A concern with quality shapes the content of management dashboards, service reviews, many payment and reward systems, and various forms of health service competition and marketing activity. 'Quality' often remains undefined, but it is so influential in healthcare systems that it warrants careful critical consideration.

In this chapter we examine the concept of 'healthcare quality', paying particular attention to the normative implications of the invocation of quality, and the use of list-like quality definitions. The chapter starts by considering how the meaning of 'quality' in healthcare relates to the meaning of 'good healthcare', highlighting the somewhat technical meaning that quality has acquired within healthcare policy, health services management and healthcare improvement, and its association with approaches to healthcare improvement that rely heavily on measurement. We then look in more detail at why quality is widely taken to be multidimensional and discuss some influential multidimensional specifications of healthcare quality. We argue that quality is best understood to be plural not only because it has several aspects but also because it means different things in different contexts and depending on improvement purposes. We explore how to approach questions about what counts as 'better' or 'worse' quality when there are diverse and potentially competing considerations at stake. Finally, while recognizing the pragmatic value of more schematic and technical approaches to specifying and measuring dimensions of quality for improvement purposes, we draw attention to their limitations and ethical implications including some of the potential pitfalls to be considered in their use.

Accounts of 'healthcare quality' rest upon assumptions and arguments about what healthcare is for and what good healthcare looks like. This, we argue, means that rather than thinking that the meaning of 'healthcare quality' must be determined *before* healthcare can be evaluated, defining healthcare quality already requires evaluative judgements. While a definition of quality can help people make practical assessments of whether healthcare is good, or is getting better, it will always reflect and promote a particular vision of good healthcare. One upshot of this is that there is not much sense in searching for an account of quality that reflects an ultimate truth about good healthcare. Would-be improvers would do better to think carefully about what good healthcare looks like – or *should* look like – in their context and for their purposes and those of other system stakeholders, in order to develop context-appropriate characterizations of quality.

3.1 What is healthcare quality?

In ordinary everyday language, 'good quality healthcare' means much the same as 'good healthcare'. Patients and members of the public are likely to take a question about the quality of a health service to ask much the same as a question about how good a health service is. (We revisit this common-sense usage in the final section of this chapter.) But it is important to recognize that, in healthcare contexts, quality has acquired a somewhat specialized meaning. When healthcare organizations, healthcare professionals and health service researchers talk about healthcare quality they often identify a list of attributes that healthcare organizations should aim to have: quality healthcare is safe, effective, caring and so on. Before looking at the lists themselves, we begin with more general exploration of the concept of healthcare quality and how it relates to these characteristics.

There is a notable duality in the meaning of 'quality'. The word 'quality' can mean a degree of excellence, but it can also refer, more neutrally, to a characteristic or a characterization of what something is like, without necessarily implying an evaluation of how good or bad it is. There is, then, both an explicitly *normative* interpretation of 'quality', which reflects how good something is or how it compares to other relevant examples, and a more *descriptive* interpretation, which reflects the features or properties that something has. Many accounts of healthcare quality elide these two senses of quality and identify a number of characteristics, the presence of which indicates good healthcare. The World Health Organization (WHO), for example, specifies that quality healthcare should be 'effective', 'safe' and 'people-centred'.[2] Accounts such as this are descriptive, insofar as they pick out qualities or features that healthcare systems can have, and normative, insofar as they indicate that healthcare systems *should* have these characteristics. We will argue that, given the way that lists of quality dimensions are used in practice, their normativity needs to be clearly recognized.

While it is common for a list of 'dimensions' of healthcare quality to be talked about as though it *is* healthcare quality, as though the dimensions themselves make up or constitute quality, the dimensions are perhaps better understood to be objectives or aims against which 'quality' is assessed. On this understanding, quality is a more holistic or multifaceted judgement of healthcare value. Healthcare quality, we suggest, is best understood as the degree to which a healthcare system or service achieves desired objectives or possesses desired characteristics. Some attempts to define quality – rather than specify quality dimensions – reflect this understanding. The Institute of Medicine in the United States, for example, has defined quality of care as 'the degree to which health services for individuals and populations increase the likelihood of desired health outcomes and are consistent with current professional knowledge' and the Council of Europe as the degree to which the treatment dispensed increases the patient's chances of achieving the desired results and diminishes the chances of undesirable results, having regard to the current state of knowledge.[3] These definitions of quality talk about 'desired' and 'undesired' outcomes or results but don't go a long way towards specifying what those desired results are, or by whom they are desired. It is the 'dimensions' of quality which provide the specification for healthcare quality. Many definitions of healthcare quality also provide a more detailed explication of the characteristics in question – defining what 'safe' or 'effective' means in practice, specifying to what extent a healthcare system needs to exhibit or pursue these ideals, and sometimes stipulating indicators and metrics. While these specifications can look quite technical in nature, they retain their normative component – that is, they say something about what form healthcare and healthcare systems *should* take.

Thus understood, 'healthcare quality' involves some kind of operational definition and specification of, or benchmark for, good healthcare systems and services. Many characterizations of quality have a structure similar to the WHO account mentioned above – insofar as they specify a number of aims or desirable characteristics of healthcare systems – but they may include different or additional dimensions. Assessing healthcare quality is, on this picture, a matter of determining whether and to what extent healthcare has the specified characteristics, and healthcare quality improvement involves introducing these characteristics or increasing their extent. Often such assessments and improvements will refer to specific indicators and metrics which represent and give substance to the more general headline dimensions.

We have begun to set out in broad brushstrokes how the idea of 'healthcare quality' is talked about and used. Hopefully it is already becoming clear that, while healthcare quality is closely related to the idea of 'good' healthcare, it typically reflects a particular way of thinking about and assessing good healthcare, namely a schematic approach which sets out key aims or characteristics and determines the extent to which they are met. The ambiguity in the very idea of quality – that it can refer to a characteristic that something can have *and* a conception of excellence against which something can be judged – means that the normative role that is played by discourses of quality in healthcare improvement can become obscured. As already noted, it is easy to slip into the assumption that a characterization of relevant evaluative dimensions provides an account of what quality is, as a matter of fact. This background assumption can be reinforced by use of specified indicators and metrics which add to the sense that quality is a definite *thing* that can be identified and defined. It is important to be aware of this risk of reification through which a broad evaluative framework is turned into an object, or by which, roughly speaking, an adjectival expression like 'better healthcare' can be transformed into a noun, 'quality'. This process enables, and is then reinforced by, an influential role for specific technical ways of knowing.[4]

The language of 'quality' in healthcare, and the schematic approach that this represents, can partly be explained by its historical roots in the twentieth-century 'quality movement' in manufacturing industry. At its most basic, 'quality' in manufacturing means conforming to an operational specification – if a car or a pair of jeans meets the specification then it will pass 'quality control'. Walter Shewhart's 'statistical process control' method from the 1920s was an early example of a quality control process which went beyond merely auditing and checking products for defects, and instead used statistical methods to monitor trends in defects and variation – for example how variation increases with seasonal changes in temperature, humidity or resources, or as machinery wears down over time.[5] This ensured that problems could be identified early or even before they arose and allowed for continual adjustment of processes to ensure sufficiently standardized outputs.

Subsequently, quality control processes were refined, developed and spread internationally, including by W. Edwards Deming, who popularized what became known as the 'Plan–Do–Check–Action' (PDCA) cycle, an approach that involves modifying existing processes to address problems and monitoring the effects to generate incremental improvements.[6] Quality control methods such as Total Quality Control, Total Quality Management, Lean and Six Sigma were developed and deployed in efforts to reduce waste and variation, improve productivity and promote efficiency on production lines. New Public Management approaches to organizing and delivering public services, introduced in the 1980s and 1990s, adopted some of these industrial methods in efforts to make public sector organizations and services – including healthcare services and systems – more 'business-like' and evidence-based in their management and operational practices.[7] Measurement and improvement of the processes and outcomes of public services and attempts to minimize waste and cut slack in their systems were central to these endeavours. The language of 'quality' and 'quality improvement' was used in service sectors – as it had been in manufacturing contexts – to characterize and manage the desirable outputs and outcomes of public services.

The dominant account of 'healthcare quality' that has emerged from this context has three distinctive characteristics:

First, it involves specification of good practice. That is, references to 'quality' typically signify some attempt to set out the aims and objectives of healthcare, and to provide some detail as to what it would look like to do it well. This might include an account of what level of variation is acceptable, or a designation of a minimum 'floor' representing the level at which performance or outcomes can be considered satisfactory. Healthcare systems are liable to have rather more – and more complex and contested – aims and objectives than industry, in part because they perform a great deal of different services and procedures, and often on human beings, but also because they typically serve a public function. This means that 'good' healthcare will be responsive not just to subjective experiences and what individual patients want, as 'customers' or 'clients' of the system, but also to considerations of broader social and political goods and values, as well as theoretical and applied knowledge of physiology, anatomy, pathology, pharmacology and so on.

Second, in this account, measurement and decision-making based on measurement are central to understanding healthcare quality. The value of measurement in healthcare decision-making has been recognized since at least the mid-nineteenth century, when Florence Nightingale demonstrated that the hospital admissions she studied led to higher mortality.[8] Measurement can enable people to see things that cannot be apprehended by direct observation. It can help overcome some of the limitations of individual perspectives, because it can provide a more detached or 'objective' representation of systems and support the development of aggregated information and recognition of patterns over time. Measurement has become normalized and increasingly obligatory in healthcare decision-making. The idea that 'you can't manage what you can't measure' is often associated with the quality movement, which seeks to ensure that assessments about how well systems are functioning are based on clear evidence. The basic idea is simple: if improvers make a claim about how good or bad a healthcare system or process is, and what should be done to change things, they need to be able to point to features which justify their assessment. This is easier said than done as, in practice, there is liable to be disagreement about the validity and reliability of measures, and evidence may be inconclusive if systems are good in some respects and not others.

Third, healthcare quality is action guiding. Defining and assessing healthcare quality is not just an academic or reporting exercise but is done with the purpose of bringing about desired outcomes. Definitions and models of healthcare quality are used to improve measured healthcare quality, averting deterioration in measured variables, or identifying and preventing unacceptable variation in care. To this end, healthcare quality is often linked with the use of improvement tools and techniques. The link with industrial quality control has furnished the practice of healthcare quality assessment and quality improvement with a number of tools and approaches, which reflect particular techniques for systematically measuring, incrementally changing and – all being well – improving healthcare systems and processes. These techniques allow for interventions to be implemented and their outcomes to be recorded methodically. This enables independent assessment and replication of quality assessment and improvement activities, generating information which researchers, policymakers and practitioners can harness to scale successful activities, design widely applicable interventions and make more generalizable claims to drive more and faster healthcare improvement. Quality assessment and improvement tools and techniques thus facilitate – at least in theory – the action-guiding application of healthcare quality.

We emphasized above that the invocation of healthcare quality represents one way of thinking and talking about good healthcare which reflects a particular set of ways of knowing. 'Quality' talk puts an emphasis on structured specifications of good healthcare, including the specification of dimensions and of the evidence-base and justification needed to make claims about good healthcare. While there is much to be said in favour of such a structured approach, it also has important limitations, including a tendency to mask normativity, which we will say more about towards the end of this chapter.

3.2 Healthcare quality is multidimensional

So 'quality' in healthcare is used to represent some kind of specification or benchmark for good healthcare systems and services. As suggested above, healthcare quality is widely regarded as multidimensional. This means that it cannot be adequately described in terms of a single characteristic or property and is instead seen to be made up of a number of different irreducible aspects or 'dimensions'. Those working in healthcare improvement will be familiar with mainstream multidimensional characterizations of healthcare quality. The US Institute of Medicine (IOM) account, introduced in Chapter 1, which is very widely used and adapted, characterizes healthcare quality in relation to six aims: healthcare should be (1) safe, (2) effective, (3) patient-centred, (4) timely, (5) efficient and (6) equitable.[9] In this section, we say a bit more about what multidimensionality is and why quality is taken to be multidimensional.

Many concepts in the social sciences are understood to be multidimensional. Naming a number of different dimensions helps to set out and specify complex concepts with a degree of clarity and precision; it also helps to make indefinite concepts more amenable to measurement by characterizing them in more definite terms.[10] We suggest that the multidimensionality of healthcare quality plays three distinct roles, which relate to the three characteristics of healthcare quality described in Section 3.1. First, it plays a conceptual role, by reflecting, and going some way towards specifying, some of the complexity of healthcare systems and what it takes for them to be 'good'. Second, it helps to make healthcare quality measurable, by providing an initial level of specification that enables more detailed operational definitions and measures of healthcare quality. And third, it supports practical-ethical decision-making, by representing the areas that should be prioritized in health policy and decision-making about healthcare system design, resource allocation and improvement activity. We will explore each of these roles in a little more detail.

First, multidimensional characterizations of quality set out the key functions and features of healthcare systems. The IOM specifies six dimensions (safe, effective, patient-centred, timely, efficient, equitable), the WHO specifies three (safe, effective, people-centred) and England's National Quality Board specifies seven (safe, effective, responsive and personalized, caring, well-led, sustainably resourced, equitable).[11] In setting out a variety of dimensions these accounts say something about the variety of things that healthcare systems do and how they should do them. The dimensions point to aspects of healthcare that go beyond clinical and biomedical processes and outcomes – if healthcare should be judged not just on how effective and safe it is, but also on how caring, timely and responsive it is to patients, this reflects a concern with people's lives more broadly, and not just their narrowly defined health states. The different dimensions also reflect that healthcare systems are complex social systems with a number of different functions. Some dimensions primarily reflect concern with treatment of and outcomes for specific patients (effective, people-centred, caring), whereas others reflect health system- or population-focused values (efficient, equitable, sustainably resourced). In this way, offering a multidimensional characterization – rather than solely focusing on a single specific aspect of healthcare, such as clinical effectiveness, for example – can give a more nuanced and realistic account of the nature and scope of healthcare systems.

Second, classifying the dimensions of healthcare quality can be the first step towards other forms of representation and measurement, including further specification of indicators and metrics. The concepts of 'good', or 'bad', or 'good quality' healthcare are relatively thin ethical concepts.[12] This means that, while they provide a normative evaluation of the healthcare in question, they don't say anything very substantive about it – the ways in which it is good or bad, for example, and what properties or characteristics form the basis of this assessment. The specified dimensions of healthcare quality are typically *thicker* ethical concepts. A thick ethical concept comprises both a normative evaluation and a description of the ways in which it is good or bad. When healthcare is assessed to be safe, or timely, or equitable, an evaluation is made of it as good, but the sense in which it is good is also narrowed down – a safe process or action is good in some more-or-less definite respects. Of course, a headline thick ethical concept like 'safe' or 'equitable' still provides relatively little detail. As we will discuss more fully in Chapters 4 and 5, there are many, sometimes competing, ways of fleshing out quality dimensions in practice. But even so, their labels and introductory descriptive content provide a basis for further specification and measurement which is comparatively absent from thin ethical concepts.

Third, multidimensional characterizations support practical-ethical decision-making. The multidimensional specification picks out certain characteristics but does not set out everything that a healthcare system does or all of the ways in which it can be good or bad. If they are well-conceived, the dimensions will reflect what are reasonably and widely taken to be important characteristics and priorities of healthcare systems or services. These judgements have both pragmatic and normative aspects. On the one hand, the selection reflects a pragmatic strategy – for healthcare quality to be a useable and operationalizable concept, it must be selective and limit the number of features that it focuses on. On the other hand, the selection reflects a normative strategy – that is, a given specification of healthcare quality picks out and emphasizes things that those making the selection take to matter most, for example because they consider them to be core features of healthcare that have been relatively overlooked in the past and need to be given precedence now. As Avedis

Donabedian, a physician and public health specialist who was an early advocate of measuring and assessing the quality of healthcare, puts it: 'the definition of quality … is, ordinarily, a reflection of the values and goals current in the medical care system and in the larger society of which it is a part'.[13] In this way, specifying a limited set of dimensions can help improvers to focus on key goals and attend to the things which matter most.

3.3 Healthcare quality is radically plural

We have argued that the idea of healthcare quality is typically used to describe a more structured, often technical, approach to thinking about and specifying good healthcare as multidimensional. In this section we say more about what the dimensions of healthcare quality are and how different, and potentially inconsistent, high-level specifications of quality should be understood in relation to one another. We argue that quality is not just plural in the sense that it is multidimensional, but more radically plural, in the sense that different context- and purpose-specific specifications of quality can reasonably be used and defended alongside one another.

Despite broad agreement about the multidimensionality of healthcare quality, the dimensions themselves are not agreed upon. We have already noted several different characterizations of quality, and these represent only the tip of the iceberg. Beyond the small number of accounts that are widely used, many national and international healthcare systems and bodies take it upon themselves to develop their own characterizations of healthcare quality – and sometimes more than one over several years or decades. Many of these identify some of the same, or similar, dimensions, but there are notable differences between them too.

The three examples we have already given are a good place to start to illustrate the overlaps and divergences between different characterizations of the dimensions of healthcare quality (see Table 1).

There are clearly similarities between these three lists. All three organizations agree that healthcare systems should be safe and effective. All three also show a concern for person-centredness or responsiveness to the needs and preferences of patients, although this is slightly differently

Table 1 Three Prominent Quality Definitions

Institute of Medicine (2001)	World Health Organization (2018)	National Quality Board (2021)
Safe	Safe	Safe
Effective	Effective	Effective
Patient-centred	People-centred	Responsive and personalized
Timely	And *in order to realize the benefits of quality healthcare' health services must be:*	Caring
Efficient	Timely	Well-led
Equitable	Equitable	Sustainably resourced
	Integrated	Equitable
	Efficient	

Sources: Institute of Medicine (2001); World Health Organization (2018); National Quality Board (2021).[14]

expressed in each case ('patient-centred', 'people-centred' and 'responsive and personalised'). The similarities indicate that accounts of healthcare quality can have much in common, at least at a very general level. But there are also clear differences. The NHS includes 'caring' and 'well-led' as dimensions, which are not listed by the others. The WHO treats 'timely', 'efficient' and 'equitable' not as dimensions of quality but as necessary enabling factors, whereas the IOM treats these as dimensions of quality. The WHO also includes 'integrated' as an enabling factor, a concept not explicitly covered in the other characterizations. Looking more closely at the definitions provided by each organization for each dimension reveals further similarities and differences. The NHS dimension of 'sustainably-resourced' includes something like 'efficiency' but goes beyond this to also include a focus on reduced adverse impacts on public health and the environment. The IOM and WHO have almost identical definitions of 'safe' care, emphasizing the need to avoid iatrogenic harm – harm that is caused by medical treatment or procedures. The NHS, by contrast, uses a rather more demanding and specific definition of safe care: 'delivered in a way that minimizes things going wrong and maximizes things going right; continuously reduces risk, empowers, supports and enables people to make safe choices and protects people from harm, neglect, abuse and breaches of their human rights; and ensures improvements are made when problems occur'. More generally the longer definitions of each dimension indicate differences in emphasis, even where the same headline word is used to describe the dimension.

These three organizations represent different national and international contexts and potentially quite different purposes. It is also worth noting the variety of characterizations of quality dimensions that can co-exist within a given context. In England, for example, other multidimensional accounts of healthcare quality sit alongside the National Quality Board characterization. The Care Quality Commission (CQC), for example, is a regulatory body that centres its inspections of health and social care organizations around five questions, which represent its conception of healthcare quality:

1   Is it safe?

2   Is it effective?

3   Is it caring?

4   Is it responsive to people's needs?

5   Is it well-led?[15]

The Health and Social Care Act (2012) in England sets out a statutory duty for the Secretary of State for Health to improve quality of services, in particular in relation to outcomes showing:

1   The effectiveness of the services;

2   The safety of the services; and

3   The quality of the experience undergone by patients.[16]

Again, there are clear similarities and differences between these accounts – all emphasize safety and effectiveness, for example, and the CQC overlaps with five out of the seven National Quality Board dimensions. This similarity is perhaps unsurprising as the CQC is one of the organizations represented on the National Quality Board. The absence of some of the National Quality Board dimensions from the CQC and Health and Social Care Act (2012) accounts of quality may reflect the perceived lower importance of dimensions such as 'caring', and 'sustainably resourced'. But it could also reflect an increased awareness of the importance of other dimensions over time – the Act was passed in 2012, the CQC 'five questions' were first launched in 2013[17] and the

National Quality Board published its first version of characterization of quality in 2016.[18] Regardless, all these characterizations of quality operate simultaneously, in broadly the same context, although they are used by different organizations for different purposes.

One way of thinking about what is going on here is to think of each of the different characterizations of healthcare quality as aiming to provide a universal and correct definition of healthcare quality. In that case, the differences between them would indicate that most – or perhaps all – of them have got it wrong, and all organizations who want to use the concept of healthcare quality should be trying to alight on the same, correct characterization. We don't see this as a helpful way to think. Each characterization of healthcare quality is developed in a particular context and for particular purposes, and each reflects a particular set of goals, aims and values. This goes a long way to explaining the divergences between them. It also suggests that each characterization could be good in some contexts and for some purposes. Some differences may be relatively arbitrary or accidental, perhaps reflecting particular 'policy moments' or the preferred jargon of influential actors, but it is also possible to interpret the divergences as intentional products of reasonable thought. This suggests that quality is not only multidimensional, but also plural in a more radical way, which might be called 'competitively plural'.[19] That is, the meaning of 'quality' is subject to variation, and sometimes disagreement, that arises from different vantage points and perspectives. Different high-level conceptions of quality can be appropriately invoked in different contexts and serve different purposes.

Sometimes the contextual and pragmatic nature of characterizations of healthcare quality is explicit in the way quality is defined and discussed. The IOM, for example, explains: 'The committee proposes six aims for improvement to address key dimensions in which today's healthcare system functions at far lower levels than it can and should.'[20] This indicates that the quality dimensions it sets out are responsive to a particular point in time and set of problems. The National Quality Board's 'shared commitment to quality' 'provides a nationally agreed definition of quality'.[21] Even this is not intended as a universal definition, however, but instead developed to enable better coordinated leadership between national bodies in England. A shared account of quality in this case serves pragmatic purposes, rather than aiming at something like conceptual truth.

Characterizations of healthcare quality, we are arguing, are best understood to be a function of the needs and purposes of particular health systems and organizations, and should not be seen as exhaustive. That is, the dimensions of quality shouldn't be understood to reflect every characteristic that is relevant to good healthcare. Rather, the stated dimensions can serve to highlight healthcare priorities and emphasize values that their advocates consider important or historically overlooked. The fact that some dimensions are missing from some characterizations of quality does not mean that the people who construct or select the characterizations of quality see these components as irrelevant to good healthcare – just that they do not take them to be core priorities for the system or organization at the time the characterizations are made. This does not mean that characterizations cannot be criticized as being unsuited to their intended context and role nor that there are no important omissions. Some important aspects of healthcare may be left out of accounts of healthcare quality because they are overlooked, rather than as a consequence of careful reasoning.

Seeing accounts of healthcare quality as pragmatic and contextual can bring into focus their limitations, as well as the ways in which they serve valued ends. One aspect of healthcare systems that is routinely left out of characterizations of quality, for example, is delivering healthcare services in ways that reflect the rights, well-being and professional integrity of employees. Such considerations might sometimes be subsumed under other dimensions; for example, employee- or staff-centredness and workforce well-being might be seen to come within an expansive conception of 'person-centredness'. But sometimes, and particularly when there is a perceived need to prioritize previously overlooked aspects of healthcare, it might be wise to highlight these neglected concerns by treating them as a separate dimension of quality in their own right. Specifying 'employee-centred' as a core dimension of quality might, for example, facilitate its being seen as a strategic priority, enabling resources to be allocated to projects that seek to improve the training and working conditions for healthcare professionals and to prioritize these concerns vis-à-vis other important concerns. Even if employee-centred healthcare is valued in large part for instrumental reasons, including the benefits it can bring to other quality dimensions such as safety and person-centred care for patients, labelling it as a quality dimension in its own right might be justified as a means to support improvement in these other domains.

If characterizations of healthcare quality reflect different purposes and ends, then healthcare quality is multiply specifiable and realizable. There is not a single, best account of what healthcare quality means or comprises. Rather, in order to know how best to understand healthcare quality, improvers need to pay attention to the healthcare context that they are working in and the reasons that they are trying to understand healthcare quality. The idea that quality is plural means not just that there is reasonable disagreement about the meaning of quality but, more radically, that many different accounts of healthcare quality can happily co-exist. There is an indefinite number of possible dimensions and combinations of dimensions of quality and, while there are of course important similarities between different health services and systems, the factors that are priorities for one context may not be priorities everywhere, because of the distinct history and social setting of each health system. We suggest that the different multidimensional accounts of quality should be seen as pragmatic and heuristic tools which enable healthcare practitioners and policymakers to set out their priorities and discuss and assess healthcare systems in practice, rather than as a means of capturing the true essence of quality.

One implication of this is that the very common practice of using an existing conceptualization of quality just because other organizations have used it, or because it is widely known, may be unjustifiable in many cases. Many institutions and individuals simply use existing accounts of quality – very often the six-part IOM characterization – even though they were explicitly developed with the aims and requirements of a given health system at a given point in time. Substantial similarities between health systems across the world mean that a certain amount of overlap in characterizations of quality will be expected, but careful reflection is needed to ensure a good fit, and it is important to recognize that the language and emphases of some particular characterizations may reflect institutional and political contingencies which will not be relevant in all contexts. Using an older existing account of healthcare quality just because it is popular and widespread may also risk inattention to emerging issues.

3.4 Multidimensionality and deciding what is better

We have argued that different characterizations of healthcare quality and its dimensions can reflect different priorities and values. In this section, we argue that, even once improvers have settled on a particular context-appropriate characterization of healthcare quality, the meaning of quality remains contested. That is, even given a suitable overall conception of healthcare quality for a particular purpose there is very often no simple 'fact of the matter' about whether quality is getting better or worse; settling on a definition of quality does not resolve normative complexity. This contestation comes about in two important ways, which we explore in detail in this section. First, the dimensions of quality are not independent of one another: they interact in complex ways and are sometimes in tension with one another. This means that quality cannot be straightforwardly maximized by increasing performance along each dimension individually. Instead, improvers must perform balancing acts in deciding what to prioritize and when. Second, as we have already indicated, the 'same' dimension can be defined and operationalized in different ways, which will lead to different characterizations of what is 'good' and 'better' healthcare. This will involve further specification of the relationship between the dimensions as well as defining the scope, identification and measurement of each dimension. Both of these ways of specifying quality will involve normative choices and have ethical implications, which we discuss in the final section of this chapter.

3.4.1 Dimensions of quality are not independent of one another

Each component of a multidimensional concept contributes something distinctive to an understanding of it. Its meaning and value cannot be reduced to or explained in terms of the meaning and value of any of the other components. Each dimension of healthcare quality thus makes a particular contribution to any overall assessment of quality. This does not mean that each dimension is completely independent from the others, however. In practice, making changes or improvements in relation to one dimension may have knock-on effects along other dimensions.

Sometimes improvements along one dimension can go hand-in-hand with improvements elsewhere – as when improvements in patient safety also improve efficiency by reducing long hospital stays due to hospital acquired infections, for example, or by reducing rates of readmission and complications. However, sometimes the dimensions of quality can be in tension with one another, and improvements in one area can generate worse outcomes or problems elsewhere. So, for example, improving person-centredness may lead to reduced clinical effectiveness (at least when clinical effectiveness is judged on narrowly biomedical criteria), if patient preferences depart from gold standard clinical guidelines or routine treatment pathways. And increasing the timeliness or cost-efficiency of health services may compromise safety or person-centredness – additional safety checks and measures to reduce the risk of errors and adverse effects can add time to clinical interventions and cost money, as can efforts to involve patients in their care and listen to and reflect on their preferences and values about treatment options (although this latter may also save clinical time in the long run if it helps ensure treatment selections are more appropriate and patients more confident about them). The dimensions of healthcare quality will also be in tension with one another insofar as prioritizing one aspect of healthcare for improvement will use time and resources which could have been spent on other issues. While these opportunity costs do not represent conceptual conflicts between the dimensions, it is important to recognize that in practice it is rarely, if ever, possible to pursue all aims and values simultaneously in resource constrained environments.

The existence of tensions between dimensions of healthcare quality means that quality cannot be increased or maximized simply by increasing or maximizing performance along each dimension. Instead, assessing and improving quality can involve making trade-offs between different dimensions – accepting less of one thing of value in order to achieve something else. Sometimes it will be reasonable and justified to accept a worse outcome along one dimension in order to secure a substantial improvement elsewhere; sometimes the cost will be considered too great. Assessing and improving healthcare quality overall therefore involve balancing different goods, and deciding which achievable combinations represent better outcomes.

This suggests that quality shouldn't be treated as a property of health systems that can be observed, but rather an evaluative assessment that is grounded in other properties and assessments. The same broad characterization of the dimensions of healthcare quality can lead to quite different assessments of healthcare quality and quality improvement in practice, depending on how dimensions are specified, which trade-offs are made and what the optimal combinations of goods are thought to be. Balancing the different dimensions of healthcare quality – and, importantly, doing it *well* – is likely to look quite different across different social and temporal contexts, which will involve different budgets, workforce and resources as well as different legal requirements and conventional expectations about the provision of healthcare.

3.4.2 Dimensions of quality can be defined and combined in different ways

The way that the dimensions of quality are fleshed out in detail will influence broader evaluative claims about healthcare quality. Underlying any assessments of healthcare quality are a number of other decisions and claims about the relationship between the dimensions of quality, their scope and how to identify their presence and absence in practice. We briefly outline three clusters of decisions which are involved in operationalizing quality dimensions: (a) the relative importance of the dimensions; (b) their scope and broad character; (c) the indicators, metrics and data sources used to make assessments of actual or predicted health system functioning.

First, then, knowing a list of the three or five or seven dimensions of healthcare quality that have been identified for a particular social or institutional context does not itself reveal anything about the relative importance of the different dimensions. It might be that they all have equal importance and should be given equal weighting in decisions. Or it could be that one or some of the dimensions are more important than others – in times of crisis or severe budgetary constraint, it might be permissible to cut corners in some areas but not others. Or perhaps small deficits in some areas may be acceptable in order to secure moderate gains elsewhere. The relative weighting of dimensions of healthcare quality could be temporary or permanent. So, for example, a team of improvers could, in principle, determine that safety is always more important than timeliness, and safety procedures should never be skipped in order to meet time-related targets. Or, similarly, they could decide that considerations of equality have been systematically overlooked in decision-making in their team, institution or wider context in recent years or decades and therefore they should prioritize these considerations in assessments of quality until the balance has been somewhat redressed.

Second – as briefly illustrated in Section 3.3 and as we discuss more fully in Chapters 4 and 5 – there are different ways of broadly characterizing each of the dimensions of quality, which will result in quite different accounts of 'good' and 'better' healthcare. One example of this is the difference between 'Safety-I' and 'Safety-II' as alternative conceptions of safety as a dimension of healthcare.[22] Safety-I reflects a more traditional conceptualization of patient safety in which safe healthcare is healthcare which largely avoids medical care or treatment causing preventable physical harm to patients. Safety-I might emphasize preventing instances of medical error and adverse events, such as hospital acquired infections; wrong side, wrong procedure and wrong patient surgeries; and mistakes in prescription or dosage. When things go wrong, efforts would be made to track the cause of the error, determine if and how it could have been avoided, and take steps to prevent (as far as possible) a repeat of the error. A Safety-I approach might advocate greater standardization of processes and procedures, and reduction of variation in performance and outcomes. Safety-II, by contrast, emphasizes success and good performance rather than failure. A Safety-II characterization of safety might focus on the ways that healthcare professionals achieve successful outcomes in dynamic environments, adapting to treat patients with different histories and needs, work with different colleagues, and respond to a demanding, constantly changing and unpredictable context. A Safety-II approach is more likely to identify the adaptive behaviours that healthcare professionals exhibit to respond effectively to unexpected circumstances, rather than try to ensure that they always conform to standardized and specified guidelines. While both of these conceptions are broadly capturing something about safe care, the way that they frame this is very different, and as a consequence the specific indicators of it and ways of measuring and identifying it will be highly divergent.

Another example of two different ways of conceptualizing a dimension of quality is the difference between more narrowly biomedical and broader biopsychosocial accounts of clinical effectiveness. A biomedical conception of effectiveness might broadly see effective healthcare as curing disease, correcting physiological abnormalities, extending length of life or otherwise achieving the kinds of ends stereotypically associated with medical practice and the ends of healthcare institutions. Biomedical perspectives on effectiveness could involve emphasizing the clinical success of surgeries and interventions, eradication of infection and infectious disease, avoidance of readmission and relief or elimination of symptoms. A biopsychosocial account of effectiveness might, by contrast, emphasize a wider range of shorter- and longer-term outcomes of healthcare, including patients' experiences of encounters with staff and other processes, and the implications for what matters in their lives, including their emotional well-being. If an intervention is biomedically successful (in removing a tumour, for example, or reducing the level of a blood marker associated with a risk of stroke) but leaves a patient distressed or even traumatized, or does not improve their health-related well-being, it might be thought, on a biopsychosocial model, to be relatively ineffective. Biopsychosocial accounts of effectiveness might also pay attention to the broader impact of medical care: a course of antibiotics which clears up an infection but is part of a prescribing policy which contributes to anti-microbial resistance would likely be considered ineffective in a broader sense, despite its being narrowly biomedically effective. In both of these examples, the way that safety and effectiveness are defined has implications for their scope and will likely lead to quite distinct assessments of good healthcare. The broad characterization of a dimension of quality will have knock-on effects for the indicators, metrics and data sources that can be used to make claims about it.

Third, in order to make assessments of any dimension of healthcare quality, improvers need to be able to identify whether it is present and to what extent. That is, for practical purposes within an institutional context, they need to operationalize each dimension such that they can say, with some degree of confidence, whether and when some instance of healthcare or some healthcare system is safe, caring, well-led and so on. To do this they will need to first identify some of the *indicators* for each dimension, that is, the features of healthcare which denote high or low performance for each dimension. Different indicators can be picked out to represent broadly the same dimension, depending on how its nature and scope is conceived. So, person-centredness in general practice might be indicated by efforts by healthcare professionals to understand a patient's preferences, values and emotional needs, by involvement of patients in significant decisions about their care, or by the continuity of care between healthcare professionals and institutions. These indicators capture different aspects of person-centred care, and emphasis on different sets of indicators can reflect a different broad conceptualization of person-centredness.

Operationalizing a dimension of quality will also involve the identification of *metrics* to determine the degree to which each indicator is present in a healthcare service or practice. Identifying metrics will enable standardized assessment of the presence or absence of each indicator, so that comparison can be made across different patients or different instances of care. So, for example, the involvement of patients in significant decisions might be measured via evidence of the use of shared decision-making tools, by an assessment of whether patients felt involved in decisions about their care, by an assessment of whether the healthcare professional felt that they had involved patients in decisions, or by evidence of consent by patients for medical treatment and interventions. Measures can be quantitative or qualitative, but they must enable comparison between different services or instances of care, such that it can be said which has more or less of the relevant indicator, or whether they are on a par. Some form of measurement is necessary for reliably and accurately assessing healthcare quality and its dimensions – without this, improvers would have descriptive claims about what would be better or worse, but limited tools for comparing or evaluating healthcare in practice.

Finally, operationalization involves the identification of *data* sources. Measuring the achievement of indicators might draw on clinical records, experience surveys, trial data, observational data and so on. Depending on the indicators and metrics chosen, different data sources will be appropriate, though there may be more than one possible dataset which can be used to measure the same thing. The choice of data source will likely be largely pragmatic, depending on the time and resources available, what kind of an assessment is being made, existing available data, technological equipment and expertise and other contextual factors. But the choice of dataset can also reflect more substantive values – collecting and seeking to understand the views of patients on their care, for example, can reflect a concern with and respect for them as participants in healthcare, rather than just passive recipients of it.

Making assessments of healthcare quality and its constitutive dimensions involves a great number of operational decisions. There is unlikely to be an obvious or single correct choice for each of these decisions, and choices may reflect a compromise between ideal and practicable options. Typically, choices will reflect and promote distinct value sets, whether this is explicit or implicit in reasoning and decision-making or not. However, the way that the meaning of dimensions and the indicators, metrics and data sources are considered and identified, as well as the approach to weighting and trade-offs between quality dimensions which shape claims about healthcare quality and quality improvement, can be thoughtful and reflective or relatively unplanned and unthinking. Reflective consideration of these factors will enable quality assessments that are context appropriate and it may also facilitate awareness of the limitations of what assessments express about healthcare practice. If the operationalization of quality and its dimensions is not reflective – if indicators and measures are settled on without consideration of the value judgements they embody or alternative possibilities – then assessments of quality risk making exaggerated claims or overlooking the shortcomings and contextual nature of resulting assessments of quality.

Regardless of whether this process is managed carefully or not, different definitions of the dimensions of quality – not only at the level of broad initial description but also at an operational level – will generate different quality assessments and different judgements relating to improvement. That is, different specifications will generate different accounts of what is 'good' and 'better'. This means that characterizations of quality not only involve normative commitments and judgements insofar as the selection of dimensions reflects particular values and priorities but making them operational and deploying them also has normative implications. If the implicit normativity of such judgements is not recognized and made explicit, there is limited opportunity to check whether the values and priorities in question are justified or judged appropriate by those who are affected by them. When quality is operationalized, what ends up being measured, and so what contributes to assessments of healthcare quality, is inevitably a relatively narrow set of factors. This doesn't mean that it fails to express anything about good and better healthcare – the specification and operationalization of quality may helpfully elucidate important aspects of the performance of a healthcare system – but it does mean that it offers just one of many possible schemata for thinking about good healthcare. It is crucial for those involved in healthcare quality assessment and quality improvement to be aware of the limitations of their conception of quality, and the ways in which it could have been or could be different.

3.5 Normative implications of thinking about good healthcare in terms of 'quality'

We started this chapter by considering the relationships between 'healthcare quality' and 'healthcare quality improvement', on the one hand, and just 'good healthcare' and 'healthcare improvement', on the other. We have argued that the dominant conception of quality in the field of healthcare improvement represents one way of thinking and talking about good healthcare which reflects a particular approach to knowing and understanding. Specifically, it typically assesses healthcare against structured specifications of several dimensions of quality, emphasizes the value and role of measurement in justifying claims about good healthcare and is associated with particular tools and techniques. This concluding section explores some of the benefits and risks of framing discussions of good healthcare in terms of quality.

Constructions of quality help to turn the idea of 'good' healthcare into something that is practicably applicable and measurable within a broadly technical practical decision-making framework. The idea of 'good' healthcare is too thin to be useful for decision-makers in healthcare institutions unless it is elaborated to some extent. Quality framings do this by creating multidimensional specifications of good healthcare and standards of assessment that can be used to investigate the performance and functioning of healthcare practice and systems. Invoking healthcare quality signals a pragmatic and somewhat systematic approach to thinking about good healthcare. We have argued that operationalizing healthcare quality involves making decisions about what to prioritize, what the most important aspects of good healthcare are, and how best to conceptualize and measure them.

Systematically measuring different aspects of healthcare for evidence-based decision-making can also help to call attention to some of the conflicts between different valued ends, and to clarify exactly what trade-offs need to be made. When improvers just state a list of all the key goals or dimensions healthcare, it can seem like they should be aiming for a healthcare system which maximally achieves all of these at once. However, once they start to measure whether and to what degree a healthcare system achieves these ends and start to think how it could achieve more of them, or achieve them better, it can become clear that achieving some goals will require compromises in other areas. Measuring goals and the objects of interest in healthcare systems can therefore help illuminate the trade-offs involved in assessments of quality. However, full clarity about the trade-offs depends upon recognizing and attending to the value tensions inherent in such assessments.

Up to now we have mainly been focusing on technical conceptions of quality, which are widely used in healthcare institutions but not necessarily well understood by patients and members of the public. But it is important not to lose sight of the more everyday meaning of quality. This is not unrelated to the technical usage: in ordinary language, quality means something like how good something is in comparison to other relevantly similar things, but it does not necessarily carry the implications of technical specification implicit in its usage in industrial and public sector service settings. This technical/everyday ambiguity in the meaning of quality means that it is possible to bring many different groups of people and voices into discussions of healthcare quality, but it also has the potential to produce discussions that are at cross purposes. When patients or members of the public are asked about the quality of healthcare, it is unlikely that they will refer to the quality schemas that we have been discussing in this chapter. The use of the same word and the broadly similar meaning might make it difficult for everyone to see and understand these differences – why, for instance, a patient's ideas about what could be better about a service might not be easily actionable or comprehensible if they fall outside of the operational account of quality.

Quality could be thought of as a 'boundary object' – that is, a concept which is used in different ways by different, intersecting social groups, which allows for communication between them despite different local usage.[23] A boundary object must have a common structure across all use contexts, to ensure it is recognizable and to enable translation, but it may nonetheless be employed quite differently by differently placed individuals. However, in order to make sure that those talking about healthcare quality from different perspectives understand one another, and to prevent the erasure of certain voices, it is crucial to attend to the different ways that people might use a boundary object term, and to negotiate overlapping and divergent meanings. This might involve, on the one hand, being aware of the limitations of schematic characterizations of quality and the possibility and value of thinking about good and bad healthcare outside of such framings and, on the other hand, recognizing the necessity of sometimes operating with technical specifications as an aid to practical action and well-justified decision-making.

It is worth attending to the possible risks and pitfalls associated with placing an emphasis on quality, schematically conceived, in order that they might be mitigated or avoided where possible. The dominance of the quality agenda in healthcare – where quality is largely understood in a more technical sense – can mean that other ways of thinking and learning about good healthcare and healthcare improvement are relatively sidelined. Functions and aspects of healthcare that are not so readily measurable, or whose value and measurement are highly contested, are especially prone to neglect. These include considerations or values such as solidarity and public trust, which are potentially crucial for well-functioning healthcare systems but causally complex and difficult to pursue and secure through deliberate interventions. Working with a technical quality framing might also make it difficult to capture improvements that occur not through intentional, incremental, measured change but, for example, as part of social and political movements or efforts to respond to adversity, such as war or epidemic. It would unlikely ever be justified to cause a major adverse event in order to improve healthcare or achieve some valued goals, but adversity can sometimes generate beneficial social and political change. One example of this might be the rapid developments in virtual- and telephone-based care brought into being by the COVID-19 pandemic. This is not to say that such changes should necessarily be thought to be all-things-considered improvements, but rather that they can be seen as continuous with and connected to healthcare improvement efforts, and indeed perhaps assessed in some circumstances 'as' healthcare improvements, despite not emerging from a traditional quality improvement process. It would, in theory, be possible to broaden the institutional quality agenda and see less schematic notions of good healthcare as coming under the quality umbrella, thereby cultivating a more expansive and inclusive sense of quality within official improvement discourse. However, improvers would also need to be careful that this broader agenda was not assimilated into the narrower quality agenda such that only what is measured is valued.

Operational characterizations of quality can also give the impression of universality and exhaustiveness. That is, it is easy to mistakenly assume that a particular account of healthcare quality can be transposed to any other setting, and that its dimensions reflect all and only those things that matter in healthcare. The specification of a clear and finite list of dimensions, indicators and metrics can give the impression of a comprehensive and conclusive picture of quality. This is of particular concern because a few definitions of healthcare quality remain conceptually dominant and are reproduced in many different contexts or strongly influence alternative definitions, and they are not always attended by a contextual caveat indicating the circumstances and range of setting in which they are intended to apply. Accounts of quality, as we have argued in this chapter, are evaluative claims about healthcare which can reflect particular sets of purposes and aims and emphasize particular political or institutional agendas. As such, those using operational characterizations of quality need to attend to the things that they don't capture, which may still be important even when they are not seen as institutional priorities. They also need to reflect on whether existing accounts are appropriate for their setting. Finally, and relatedly, the specification of several clearly defined dimensions of quality can make it seem like these are discrete components of quality, and that they can be dealt with largely independently. But, as we have cautioned, quality is not simply a concatenation of all its dimensions – the different dimensions of quality will inevitably interact and shape one another in complex ways. They should not be seen as discrete goals or components of healthcare systems, but as values to be emphasized or prioritized in healthcare decision-making, recognizing that it will not always be possible to pursue or prioritize every valued end in every decision.

To conclude this chapter, we briefly summarize two 'extreme' positions, both of which we think are important to resist. First, is the idea that quality should be considered as comparable to a physical property like 'length', 'mass' or 'volume' in the sense that there can be an agreed universal definition of quality that can be used as a single clear standard against which to judge whether healthcare is improving and by how much. Second, is the idea that it is sufficient to think of quality as comparable to something like 'taste' – that the diversity of quality conceptions and dimensions means that there is no reason to expect common ground about quality judgements that are wholly various and a matter of opinion. It is unlikely that anyone who has thought about healthcare quality consciously holds either of these two positions. But, we suggest, these kinds of 'pictures' can sometimes operate in the background of people's thinking and policymaking, such that, for example, they are motivated to strive towards something akin to the first picture and, in so doing, to be partly driven by anxiety about the second picture.

Something like these associations and motivations may be in play, for example, if someone is inclined to welcome and feel comfortable with the use of a quality dimension such as 'efficiency' but feels much less comfortable about a dimension such as 'person-centredness'. Efficiency may seem simply more 'solid' and clear-cut than person-centredness. Efficiency perhaps lends itself to being mathematically specified and plotted as a line on a graph. By contrast person-centredness conspicuously highlights multiple values that are in themselves somewhat indeterminate and may conflict with one another. If healthcare quality as a whole is seen as something akin to a definite property of healthcare systems, this seems to make judgements about improvement easier, and at the same time to simplify the ethics of improvement. At least, it would seem, improvers could know definitively whether their actions, whatever other complications they raise, are producing more or less improvement or quality. In this chapter we argued that this is not the right way to think about quality nor its dimensions, and that its simplification can obscure and omit something important. In the next two chapters, by focusing in on some of the most widely adopted dimensions of quality, we will develop and illustrate this argument further and expand on the discussion of the value-laden and contested decisions involved in making quality assessments. Carefully specified conceptions and operationalized measures of quality add something distinctive to the discussion and pursuit of good healthcare. However, it is important to recognize their limitations, and to acknowledge the value judgements within them and the ways that they can shape and to some extent obscure our thinking about what is good and how we can come to know it.

4 OPERATIONALIZING QUALITY

I n this chapter and the next we develop our discussion of the normative complexity of quality concepts by looking at some of the central concepts that are used to refer to dimensions of quality or aspects of good healthcare. In Chapter 3, we argued that quality is plural and that different ways of defining and specifying quality reflect different visions of the nature and scope of healthcare. The way that improvers understand quality and prioritize and balance its dimensions therefore involves a series of normative stances and choices, whether these are acknowledged or not.[1] In Chapters 4 and 5, we extend the case for recognizing that each of the designated dimensions of quality is also plural, and that their specification too involves normative or value laden judgements. This is more obvious for some dimensions (which clearly involve value choices and have contestable meanings) than for others (which appear to be more neutral and have more definite meanings). Determining what it takes for healthcare to be equitable and person-centred, for example, clearly requires consideration of individual and social attitudes and priorities, including reflection on how people should treat and relate to one another and what functions and responsibilities health services ought to have. By contrast, what it takes for a healthcare system to be effective, efficient or safe might seem to be more of a technical or bureaucratic concern than an ethical one: these dimensions seem less contestable and more determinate. The apparently 'harder' character of this second set of dimensions might suggest it contains more fixed and non-negotiable aspects of healthcare quality, compared to the first set, corresponding to relatively inflexible ways in which healthcare can be judged to be better and worse. Chapter 3 painted a picture of quality which is open-ended and contested – perhaps to an alarming extent – and this chapter explores, and ultimately rejects, the idea that harder quality concepts offer firm ground on which to build a characterization of quality.

This chapter considers putatively 'harder' quality dimensions, focusing in particular on 'efficiency' and 'safety'. One of our aims is to pause to consider these ideas in their own right to illuminate the challenges of specifying their meaning and thereby, more broadly, of characterizing what makes healthcare good and what improving it might involve. We also use these examples to argue that 'harder' quality concepts are inevitably bound up in value contests that are comparable to those routinely recognized in other more obviously value-laden areas of quality. The following chapter, Chapter 5, looks in more detail at the character of these obviously value-laden or 'softer' areas, arguing that that 'softness' reveals something fundamental about the nature of quality taken as a whole, and has substantial implications for how we should think, in both theoretical and practical contexts, about healthcare quality improvement.

The apparent 'hardness' of dimensions like efficiency and safety, we suggest, is not an inherent feature of such dimensions but something brought about by operationalization. Specifying and operationalizing quality concepts involves practical and normative decisions which reflect the goals and priorities of relevant institutions and individuals, and which can promote and endorse different values and visions of healthcare. This makes it easier to measure them and make claims about the quality and improvement of services. These are important and at times necessary aims, but it is crucial to recognize the specification and operationalization that is going on, rather than assume that 'hard' measures reflect the single best representations of the dimensions in question. Operationalization can generate a technicist façade, with clear and distinct indicators of success and failure, which masks an underlying ethical landscape characterized by nuance and uncertainty.

Towards the end of the chapter, we explore why it is important to challenge the assumption that some quality concepts are inherently more certain or stable than others. We argue that the measurement and assessment of dimensions of quality, when characterized in 'harder' ways, are well suited to decision-making which uses 'maximizing' reasoning – that is, which favours options that maximize certain pre-specified 'good' outcomes. The use of hard measures to make decisions in this way can gloss over or obscure many of the ethical tensions and choices involved in assessing quality and can give an unwarranted and potentially misleading sense of clarity.

4.1 What does operationalization involve?

It is easy to secure agreement that healthcare should be 'effective', 'efficient' or 'safe' – the value and relevance of these quality dimensions are difficult to deny. It may also be possible to agree a broad definition of them without too much trouble. But if improvers are to use these concepts to make assessments of healthcare services, they need to say more about what they mean in practice. They need to operationalize them. One way of approaching operationalization is to give examples of good and bad practice. But – to take the example of 'effectiveness' – while providing examples of effective healthcare systems can help convey a general sense of what is meant by effectiveness in a range of healthcare settings, this would be inadequate for certain purposes. In many research, management and planning contexts there is an interest in making more detailed and comparable assessments of effectiveness, and this depends upon finding some more determinate way of saying whether and why particular healthcare services are effective. To this end, improvers might stipulate the 'indicators' or features of services that make them effective or ineffective and specify any thresholds services must surpass to be considered effective. For many practical purposes it will also be necessary to explain how these indicators are to be measured, and what data and evidence (including about comparator services or population groups) to use to make claims about a service's effectiveness. For health services that aim to prevent or delay adverse outcomes, considerations of effectiveness may require assessment of time periods or rates of progression to undesirable outcomes; this will often overlap with considerations of safety and efficiency.

So, for example, operationalizing effectiveness in relation to a hospital's cardiac surgery service could include:

- identifying some key indicators of clinical effectiveness – for example, duration of post-operative survival, patient-reported quality of life, reoperation rates, post-operative infection and neurological complication rates and peri-operative death;
- determining how best to measure such indicators – for example, which clinical classification codes to use, whether to measure 'all-cause' reoperation or reoperation for bleeding, whether to

include all post-operative infections, all surgical site infections or just the most serious deep sternal wound infections, whether to use generic or cardiovascular-specific quality of life tools, and the appropriate timeframe for measuring rates of infection, stroke, heart attack and death;

- specifying what data sources and what additional evidence should be used to make and justify claims – such as routine patient records, national death registers, additional survey or data collection tools, and previous audit or research study benchmarks.

Claims about effectiveness will typically draw on some kind of comparison, for example, of how surgery's positive and negative outcomes compare with the outcomes of other kinds of treatment or no treatment. These claims will be more or less compelling depending on the quality of the data, the validity of measures, and the relevance and exhaustiveness of indicators in representing effectiveness. Our cardiac surgery example includes largely quantitative metrics, but operational specifications can also specify qualitative metrics, including of subjective experience and opinion. Developing good indicators will typically require specialist clinical, operational, statistical and/or psychometric input.

It is important to recognize that claims about effectiveness and improvement can't simply be read off data but require evaluative reflection on expectations and an understanding of good and bad practice. For example, expected and acceptable variations in outcomes must be factored into any claims about effectiveness. Moreover, changes can improve practice and outcomes in some respects and make it worse in others; assessing whether they are better overall or all-things-considered requires evaluative judgements about the relative priority of different effects. Nonetheless, the specification of quality dimensions provides us with many of the ingredients for making evaluative claims about them, even if it doesn't take us all the way to final assessments of value and improvement or ensure the truth of those claims.

Operationalizing a concept like 'effectiveness' involves specifying it in detail. But crucially operationalization also entails setting out an account of its 'epistemic conditions' – that is, explicitly specifying what it takes to be able to make knowledge claims about it, including knowing when and to what degree something is effective or ineffective (assuming that effectiveness is a concept which admits of degrees).

The epistemic conditions of features of health systems are not obvious or straightforward. This contrasts with other relatively straightforward cases. For example, knowing whether something is 'red' is usually fairly easy to ascertain, as long as the object is question in accessible to us – we look at it and make an assessment. There are disputable cases – where it is not clear whether an object is red or orange, where an object is partly but not wholly red, or where the lighting is affecting its apparent colour, for example, but our senses provide a good enough route to knowledge about many objects and entities. While it would be possible to operationalize 'redness' – and it might occasionally be necessary for certain technical tasks – it is not necessary for most colour identification purposes.

However, people can't just look at a health system or service to assess whether it is safe or effective. For one thing, a health system or service typically extends across space and time, and it is not possible for anyone to experience it in its entirety. In this way, even though a health service occurs in physical space and time, and many parts of it are experienced by different people, it is, in a sense, invisible in the same way that the economy of a nation or Christmas is invisible.[2] This is in part, as just mentioned, because these entities are too big, or temporally and spatially dispersed, to be experienced by one person, but it is also because they are conceptually indistinct. If someone says to you 'the ball is red' you will probably have a pretty good idea what the object of their claim is – the ball – which helps make it easy for you to verify the claim that it is red. If they say 'the economy is growing' or 'the health system is effective' you might well be less clear exactly what they are talking about. You might wonder where the boundaries are of these entities and what is included and excluded: whether the economy also includes black-market activities and unpaid labour, for example, and whether the health system includes private institutions or just public healthcare organizations. This makes it difficult to make confident knowledge claims about these entities without further specification.

As well as some entities being relatively indistinct and difficult to get a clear hold on, some properties are also relatively ambiguous. It is difficult to make confident knowledge claims about the 'effectiveness' of health systems or the 'growth' of the economy because these properties are relatively indistinct, compared to, say, the 'redness' of a ball. One reason for the indistinctness of properties like effectiveness and growth is related to the spatial and temporal dispersal of entities like health systems and economies – that is, if some parts of a system are effective and some parts are not, it will be ambiguous whether it is best described as effective. A second reason for the indistinctness of these properties is that their meaning is disputable and disputed. Economic growth could refer to increased Gross Domestic Product, for example, or increased Net Domestic Product.[3] Effectiveness could refer to achievement of shorter-term clinical biomedical outcomes or longer-term personal social outcomes, including well-being or social contribution. And the way these properties are defined will, in many cases, lead to different assessments.

Operationalization helps us to make knowledge claims about these complex properties of complex entities by breaking them down into more specific and manageable parts, about which less ambiguous assessments can be made, and providing a detailed specification of how the entity and the properties of interest can and, for particular purposes, should be understood. It provides a path to making specific, evidenced and justified claims about complex and contested entities. Of course, operationalization does not rule out mistakes. Knowledge claims made using the operational schema may reflect a misunderstanding or over-simplification of the entity or property under consideration. And there is, furthermore, no guarantee that a single, clear answer will emerge when using an operational specification to assess some phenomenon. Any operational specification of a complex property of a complex entity is going to involve some degree of abstraction and simplification, and, in the relevant context, this can be seen as necessary and beneficial. While something is undoubtedly lost in this process, if all goes well what is lost will be less significant than what is gained, namely a practically applicable, usable tool which allows people to make measurements and assessments in pursuit of their objectives, for example, in relation to healthcare delivery and governance. For a given quality dimension improvers can set out different possible indicators, criteria, measures and ways of acquiring evidence, and set a higher or lower bar for acceptable performance.

Some of the properties of healthcare systems seem more suited to operationalization than others. Operationalizing 'person-centredness' or 'equity', for example, is liable to be difficult because there is limited agreement about what these require in practice and their core characteristics. As we will go on to discuss in Chapter 5, different ways of describing these properties of health systems reflect and endorse different visions of healthcare, public institutions and society more broadly. Similarly, developing operational definitions to specify what it means for healthcare to be 'respectful' or 'caring' is likely to be overtly contentious because these concepts may be understood differently by different people, including different cultural and generational groups. On the other hand, some aspects of healthcare seem to be less open to discussion. What it takes for healthcare to be 'safe' for example, might not at first glance seem to be so culturally or socially inflected as other more obviously value-laden properties. It would certainly be difficult to dispute that when there are more avoidable deaths, hospital-acquired infections, prescribing errors and missed diagnoses, healthcare is less safe.

As mentioned at the start of the chapter, one way of thinking about more-easily-operationalizable aspects of quality is as 'harder' dimensions or as reflecting 'harder' outcomes. The metaphor of 'hardness' and 'softness' is sometimes used to distinguish between differences in the rigour and objectivity in measurement and knowledge claims. It is perhaps most familiar in relation to the classification of, and assertion of hierarchies within, 'hard' and 'soft' sciences. 'Hardness' is, for example, used to denote the use of controlled experiments to examine testable hypotheses, reliance on quantifiable data and mathematical modelling, metrical accuracy, high levels of consensus and replicability. 'Softness' usually denotes in-depth, localized and less generalizable studies, the use of qualitative methods, high levels of interpretation and researcher judgement throughout the research process, and often indicates the study and interpretation of the cultural rather than the physical realm.

'Hardness' and 'softness' can also be used to refer to outcomes of policies and interventions – including within healthcare improvement. A 'hard' outcome is relatively concrete or can be unambiguously defined and independently and objectively measured; it is often quantified or deemed quantifiable. A 'soft' outcome may be more intangible and measurable only indirectly; soft outcomes may also involve subjective assessment and be more obviously contested or contestable. In the context of healthcare improvement, a distinction might be drawn between relatively 'harder' research and claims relating to the (typically quantified) measurement of clinical outcomes, technical procedures, financial cost, timing and delays and relatively 'softer' (typically qualitative) research and claims relating to measures and understanding of staff and patient experience, well-being, culture and communication. Setting aside any judgement about the relative value or utility of 'hard' and 'soft' methods and measures of outcome, if these metaphors meaningfully pick out a distinction between different kinds of epistemic practice and knowledge claims, then there may be a class of healthcare improvement practices and claims which are relatively less contested and more determinate.

The relative operationalizability of some quality concepts might seem to make the plurality of quality more manageable. For it would mean that, while there remains a certain amount of contestation and variability to manage in the way healthcare quality is thought about, there are also more-or-less fixed points around which to build accounts of quality. This would help to cut through some of the indeterminacy and ambiguity with which the previous chapter ended, and so pave the way for making more generalizable and definitive claims about healthcare quality.

We think such conclusions would be misguided. We will argue that quality claims about 'harder' concepts are more ethically complex than their technical façade indicates. In the next two sections we look in detail at the examples of 'efficiency' and 'safety' in order to illustrate the ways in which they too are value-laden and relatively open-ended and to develop the argument about the benefits and costs of operationalization. We focus on efficiency and safety because, along with effectiveness, they are widely agreed to be centrally important features of healthcare quality. A closer look at some of these putatively more fixed dimensions of quality reveals that hardness is not an inherent feature of these phenomena but a useful device that helps make it easier to measure them and hold decision-makers to account. Hardness is something that is done to phenomena rather than a feature or property which they already have. Operationalizing a quality dimension in this way can close down ethical debate and uncertainty by providing a definitive specification and definition, but this serves to obscure, rather than resolve, ethical tensions and nuance.

4.2 Efficiency and operationalizing perspectives

Efficiency is very commonly invoked as a dimension of quality. Often it is used to characterize practices which seek to reduce the financial cost or resource-use of healthcare services, to cut waste or to get the most out of available resources. Efficiency can seem to be a relatively 'hard' dimension, especially when it is largely conceived in financial terms. Expenditure and use of physical resources are relatively easy to count and, when the facts and figures are assembled, identifying which of two options is cheaper, quicker or uses fewer resources may seem like a relatively straightforward task.

In this section, we argue that characterizing and assessing efficiency is a highly value-laden exercise which involves (implicitly or explicitly) defining the goals and aims of healthcare services, signalling what and who matters, and recognizing the validity of certain kinds of knowledge and information in characterizing the operation of health systems. Far from being more-or-less fixed claims about what is efficient are open to contestation, reflecting different characterizations of what matters and what healthcare service and system priorities should be. Operationalizing efficiency is, therefore, a contested activity that includes many value judgements.

Throughout this section, we draw on examples relating to home-based community healthcare services.[4] Broadly, these are primary healthcare services which involve nurses and other healthcare practitioners, with a varied skill mix, travelling to patients' homes to care for them. The care provided can include wound care, catheter and continence care, medication management and prescribing, physiotherapy, chronic disease management, essential nursing and palliative care as well as emotional or psychosocial support. Home-based care can be delivered by specialist healthcare professionals as well as generalist nurses.

4.2.1 What is efficiency?

Efficiency is an assessment of the ability of a system to maximally achieve its ends with a minimum use of resources.[5] The efficiency of all sorts of systems can be described, including mechanical and biological systems, but the concept can also be applied to the functioning of human social systems – including businesses and public institutions. Efficient systems, in all cases, are those that achieve their intended results without waste. Efficiency is widely invoked as a core dimension of healthcare quality. In assessing the efficiency of healthcare systems, the core issue is whether they could do everything they should be doing using fewer resources, or whether they could achieve more with the same resources. In principle, the resources of a healthcare system are very broad: the Institute of Medicine suggests that an efficient system avoids wasting 'equipment, supplies, ideas, and energy'.[6] But in practice a more limited range of resources are typically measured, including money, time, equipment, capacity and workforce. Similarly, while the desired ends of healthcare are in principle very varied, including knowledge, clinical outcomes, well-being and social impact, often health service efficiency is understood in terms of a quite restricted set of service-related activities, which include things like the number of visits or operations performed, workforce utilization rates and measures of bed-occupancy. The resources and ends that are typically used to characterize efficiency are ones that are relatively easy to measure.

A *technically* efficient system either achieves a defined output or end using the minimum resources or maximizes a desired output using a defined input of resources. Given a clearly defined and stable end or a fixed and defined set of resources, it becomes possible to make relatively unambiguous claims about technical efficiency. To illustrate with an example from the community healthcare context, assuming a fixed list of patients who need to be visited at home by a community nurse on a given day, the order and route can be planned so as to minimize travelling time between home visits. Depending on whether the input (time) or output (number of patient visits) as seen as fixed, a technically efficient system might either maximize the number of patient visits within a defined period or minimize the number of staff hours used to visit a defined number of patients.

However, this technical conception of efficiency is only useful for characterizing the efficiency of very simple systems, or parts of systems. Even relatively basic descriptions of healthcare services involve multiple different inputs and outputs. Healthcare services employ a range of personnel with different skills and knowledge and have a stock of equipment on which to draw. In a community healthcare service, healthcare professionals don't just visit patients, but use their skills and knowledge to meet clinical and personal needs and preferences, which potentially include patient preferences about the timing of visits and continuity of care. But as soon as a number of variables are in play, it becomes difficult to make unambiguous claims about efficiency.[7] For example, fitting the maximum number of visits into a day might involve requiring highly skilled nurses to perform basic care – thus 'wasting' their expertise – or only allowing for the most urgent care to be performed – potentially requiring subsequent visits to perform less urgent tasks. Deploying nurses in ways that make the best use of their clinical expertise might, however, require compromise on other factors such as travel time or the number of visits that can be fitted into each day, and may not be compatible with fulfilling patient preferences around continuity of care and timing of visits. Assessing efficiency in complex systems therefore requires consideration of different inputs and outputs in relation to one another.

4.2.2 Balancing and optimizing

Efficiency in complex systems, with multiple inputs and outputs, requires balancing different ends, constraints, resources and commitments. It is rarely possible to maximally achieve all the desired ends of a service with the available resources, so balancing will require trade-offs to work out how to best achieve a range of things that the relevant set of actors want the service to deliver. That is, it might be necessary to settle for slightly less of some goods or to use slightly more resources than hoped in order to achieve the range of things that the service aims to do. Whereas the more technical idea of efficiency calls for *maximizing* outputs and *minimizing* inputs, when trying to say what efficiency looks like in a system which operates with multiple different kinds of resources and tries to achieve many different ends, the focus will be on *optimizing* the set of inputs and outputs. This will involve working out what the best mix of outputs is when it is not possible to maximize all at once, or working out whether and how the use of resources such as time and money can be reduced without affecting key outputs. It may, for example, be appropriate to ask skilled nurses to perform basic care sometimes, but not all of the time, and less packed schedules could be necessary to ensure that patients have all their care needs met in one visit. There may not be a clear single most efficient (optimum) option, but rather several options which each has a credible claim to be optimally efficient because they differently satisfy an acceptably broad and balanced array of ends with reasonable and justifiable use of resources. Context-specific deliberation will be needed to decide which of these to pursue. This already starts to suggest that operationalizing efficiency is a more complex and value-laden exercise than it might seem at first, as it will require context-specific prioritization of and holistic judgements about a number of valued goods and ends, rather than a single, upfront specification of the relevant system inputs and outputs.

In order to make claims about whether a health service is efficient it is necessary to identify and define what its resources and ends are. So far, we have mainly given examples of inputs and outputs that are typically taken into account when health services think about efficiency – time, money, staff numbers and skill mix, patient numbers and needs, visits, and interventions performed. But the actual impact of health systems will extend beyond such clinical and operational outcomes; there are other, more complex, human factors which are relevant to thinking about health system efficiency, especially over the longer term. For example, fulfilment of patient preferences about continuity of care, clear communication, and the social and interpersonal benefits of care are potentially desirable ends of healthcare services. Staff retention and staff well-being could also be considered outputs of a healthcare services in their own right, as well as means to other ends. These ends are rarely prioritized in operational modelling of services and in assessments of efficiency. But it is reasonable to ask whether a health system is efficient if it achieves its clinical and operational ends within budget, but at a cost of disregarding patient preferences and experiences and staff well-being. If these personal factors are left out of operational models of efficiency, then a health service could be judged highly efficient while neglecting these important concerns.

Failure to take these more personal inputs and outputs of health systems into account could potentially be seen as inefficient both indirectly and more directly. First, these factors may have indirect long-term effects on more narrowly conceived efficiency considerations. So, for example, overworking staff and not attending to their well-being could plausibly lead to high levels of burnout and staff turnover, and services will have to bear the additional costs associated with recruitment and induction, employing temporary workers and managing staffing gaps. Burnout and staffing issues may also impact on the quality of care received by patients and their clinical outcomes, including increasing clinical errors and safety incidents. Similarly, overlooking respectful treatment, patient preferences about communication and continuity of care may result in errors of communication, leading to missed diagnoses or treatment errors, or low engagement and participation from patients, any of which could adversely affect illness experiences and clinical outcomes. Second, even if overlooking these factors does not lead to poor clinical or operational outcomes, they might nonetheless be considered to be relevant resources and ends in their own right, and so – at least in principle – suitable for consideration in an operationalized model of efficiency. It is plausibly bad in its own right, for example, if the normal functioning of healthcare systems leaves staff with substantially lower well-being, regardless of the consequences this has for patients. Health services depend on inputs such as the energy and motivation of their workforce as well as money and equipment, and staff and patient well-being are arguably desirable outputs alongside clinical and organizational outcomes.

Recognizing these less technical and more human resources and ends raises difficult questions for operationalizing efficiency: a healthcare service that achieves good outcomes for patients at the expense of staff well-being is worse, and less efficient, than one which achieves those same outcomes, using the same resources, while also protecting staff welfare. But what if maintaining staff well-being can only be achieved by settling for slightly lower patient satisfaction or clinical outcomes, or at a significant financial cost? How much of a reduction in some areas should be acceptable in exchange for gains elsewhere?

4.2.3 Efficient for whom?

Once it is recognized that a wide variety of resources and ends are potential factors to be considered in an operational model of efficiency – including personal as well as more institutional resources and ends – the ethical implications of these conflicts and trade-offs start to become clear. A decision not to include some of the more personal resources and ends in a model of efficiency, or to relatively deprioritize them vis-à-vis more institutional resources and ends, can lead to certain functions of healthcare being overlooked and key people and resources being taken for granted. So, for example, planning the daily rota in a way that does not minimize travel time, and which uses highly skilled staff to deliver basic care tasks, may seem obviously inefficient from an institutional and staff perspective. However, if the service is to prioritize continuity of care for patients and to meet their preferences about the timing of visits, and if these concerns are seen as important aims of a service, then not minimizing travel time for these reasons should be seen as at least relevant to assessing efficiency. Similarly, minimizing travel time and maximizing the number of visits a nurse can fit into each day may look like an efficient use of resources, but it may contribute to staff burnout and demoralization in the long run if, for example, it means that nurses are unable to take breaks and must repeatedly perform tasks for which they are overqualified. Not factoring the motivation and energy of staff into assessments of efficiency has the potential to overlook some of the human resources that health systems implicitly rely on, and risks labelling systems efficient when they are in fact overstretched and liable to cease being able to optimally achieve their ends.

One problem with including personal factors in operational models of efficiency is that they can be difficult to measure and can involve relatively indirect and obscure causal pathways. Working out whether and how well staffing rotas and workforce planning will efficiently deliver care which meets patients' clinical need without, for example, using highly skilled professionals to perform basic care tasks, is already an operationally difficult challenge, and requires understanding of training, skills, knowledge and capacities of health professionals as well as the range of needs of patients with different health conditions and how these are likely to change over time. Understanding how rotas and planning will efficiently deliver care that not only meets a service's clinical obligations but also satisfies patient preferences and enhances or maintains staff well-being is extremely complex. Not only is the causal relationship between a health service and these outcomes indirect and affected by other, largely external, factors, but models of efficiency might also have to draw on approaches from behavioural psychology and behavioural economics to estimate the impact of tiredness and stress on the quality of care, communication and motivation, as well as more standard operational research methods. Indeed, there may simply be no credible knowledge base to draw upon, so making confident claims about the relationship between these factors in particular contexts is likely to be difficult. All this may amount to a justification for largely keeping these factors out of assessments of efficiency, and instead looking at a more simple, technical representation of health system resources and ends.

However, if personal factors are left out of models of efficiency – and even if there is good reason to do so – it is crucial to recognize the limitations of those models, and the extent to which they will represent an institutional, and blinkered (even if knowingly blinkered), view of the function and role of health services. More generally, models of efficiency will, for practical reasons, comprise a simplified representation of health system operation.

The above discussion shows that operationalizing efficiency is not just causally complex, but also normatively complex. The factors that are included in models of efficiency will implicitly prioritize the needs and perspectives of some organizations, people and groups, and implicitly promote and endorse some values more than others. As we have indicated in the examples, the way efficiency is operationalized can overlook the impact that health services have on some people and can promote certain system functions at the expense of their health and well-being. But, in addition, it can promote certain aspects of health systems and certain ways of understanding health system function over others. If, for example, efficiency is operationalized in a hospital to minimize bed days and maximize the use of less specialized health professionals, this could end up putting a lot of pressure on the community services and primary healthcare staff to whom patients are discharged, as well as on their carers or family members. Efficiency at a service level might not, then, look very efficient at a system level, particularly if hospitals are able to deliver the care in question better or more easily than other parts of the system. Focusing on service activities and clinical outcomes rather than well-being, for example, can end up promoting a very biomedical account of the function and good functioning of health systems which may not reflect the aims of all health services, particularly those community and mental health services more adjacent to social care.

All this suggests that efficiency, far from being a relatively easy-to-measure and uncontested dimension of quality, requires searching consideration of the function and goals of healthcare, as well as attention to who healthcare systems impact on and how. The perceived 'hardness' of efficiency is largely a product of a tendency of those measuring and assessing efficiency to rely on a few, readily quantifiable resources and ends, but this is just one way of modelling efficiency, which reflects a largely institutional perspective on what healthcare systems are for and how they operate. Operationalizing efficiency depends upon choosing which factors to include in a model of the inputs and outputs of a system, and there will be range of views on what is important, which may reflect particular perspectives and purposes. Relying on those factors which have been used by others, or are commonly used in operational models of efficiency, assumes that these are the factors which are important to understanding efficiency, and overlooks other potential factors, even if this is not explicitly acknowledged. But even if it is necessary to use simplified models of efficiency for the practical purposes of assessing and comparing systems, this should be done with awareness of the models' limitations and of the important factors which are excluded from them, perhaps because they are difficult to measure or predict.

In the final section of this chapter, we will explore in more detail the potential for reductive models of quality concepts to cause problems for healthcare improvement activities, particularly when they are used without explicit attention to their limitations. But first we will discuss another example of a quality concept that is often seen as relatively 'hard', and not as widely open to interpretation as some other quality concepts: patient safety.

4.3 Safety and operationalizing harm

Safety is a pretty-well undisputed dimension of healthcare quality which focuses on the prevention of avoidable iatrogenic harm – that is, harm that is caused in the course of healthcare. 'Safety' or, as it is often labelled 'patient safety', refers to, on the one hand, an aim and outcome of healthcare – the safety of patients, and how safe patients actually are – and, on the other hand, a field of practice – the study of patient safety and activity that is oriented towards it. These two senses of safety can come apart, because patient safety research and practice may not in fact make patients safer. Traditionally, patient safety in both of these senses has been concerned with identifying and reducing the incidence of mistakes or shortfalls in healthcare practices (including prescribing errors, surgical errors, and not maintaining a sterile environment during intervention) which result in bad outcomes for patients (including adverse medication effects, bodily damage, infection and other physical harms, including death). Understood thus, safety as a dimension of quality seems like a relatively 'hard' concern: these events and outcomes are clearly bad and it is better to have less of them; moreover, it is usually possible to count them and so to assess how 'safe' care is. Safety as a healthcare priority reflects a very well-established principle of medical ethics to 'do no harm'.[8]

In this section, we consider the way that safety is often operationalized, with an emphasis on serious physical harms and relatively determinate events, and discuss how and why this represents a limited subset of possible safety concerns. We look at two questions, both gathering attention within the field of patient safety, which challenge the boundaries of this conventional construction of safety: first, asking whether 'dignitary harms' – that is, insults to a person's dignity, or injuries to their standing as a person – should be considered a patient safety concern; and, secondly, asking what safety might require above and beyond the absence of harm, including to what extent safety should be concerned with risk as well as or instead of actual harm, and the role of a safe and resilient culture in assessing safety. Overall, we show why patient safety as an aim of healthcare is less determinate than suggested by any operationalization focused on the occurrence of physical harms and how operationalizing safety is an evaluative and interpretive matter.

4.3.1 Dignitary harms

To operationalize patient safety, it is necessary to determine the scope and meaning of 'harm'. There will inevitably be contestation about what should count as a relevant harm – including which sets of physical consequences should count as harmful – but here we focus on one important area of contestation relating to what are sometimes thought about as 'psychological' factors. Specifically, some safety researchers and practitioners have argued that dignitary harms should be included within the scope of patient safety.[9] Dignitary harms are, broadly, insults to a person's dignity or moral status, caused by disrespectful or humiliating behaviour or words, which treats them as inferior. Examples of dignitary harms are hugely varied, including discussing sensitive information about a patient or their condition in public spaces, knowingly or negligently allowing patients to sit in their own excrement for extended periods of time, not referring to people by their preferred names and pronouns, ignoring patient preferences and withholding information from patients about their care. Anyone can be the subject of dignitary harms, but people who are particularly vulnerable or members of socially marginalized groups are perhaps most likely to be affected. Dignitary harms occur throughout society and are not limited to harms to patients that are caused by healthcare professionals. But disrespectful behaviour may be particularly egregious when aimed at patients, in part because healthcare professionals and institutions are supposed to help and heal patients, but also because patients are often disempowered and rendered vulnerable when healthcare environments require disclosure of sensitive information, states of undress and nakedness in semi-public settings and intimate physical contact with staff. These and other healthcare practices can make people susceptible to experiences of shame or humiliation.

Dignitary harms could fall within the scope of patient safety because they constitute indirect or direct harms. Dignitary harms can be seen as indirect harms insofar as they create the conditions in which medical errors and the kinds of major physical harm discussed above are more likely to occur. This may be because patients who are subject to disrespectful behaviour are less likely to communicate their needs and symptoms openly with healthcare professionals and may even withdraw from healthcare altogether, or because disrespectful healthcare professionals do not listen or attend to patients. Racist and sexist attitudes can manifest in false beliefs about patients, which can lead to mismanagement of pain and symptoms. So, dignitary harms can cause the kinds of physical harm which typically constitute the harms of unsafe care. But dignitary harms can also be seen as directly harmful. This is because the emotional and psychological distress and damage caused by disrespectful and humiliating behaviour is itself deemed harmful, even when it doesn't amount to serious psychiatric or physical harm.

In one study, primary care patients' self-reported the harms that they suffered in the course of healthcare, and reported 'psychological harms' far more frequently than physical or economic harms.[10] The researchers' category of 'psychological harms' included feelings of anger, frustration and belittlement, a sense of violation, diminished trust in clinicians, and anxiety about health. These are feelings and states that will likely not amount to clinical mental health issues but are nonetheless classified as harmful by patients, and which are sometimes caused by disrespectful communication and conduct by healthcare professionals. Some safety researchers have argued that harms like these should be recorded, categorized and have their severity assessed, as is currently standard with respect to physical harms.[11] Such an approach would change the standard scope of safety significantly, and assessments of the safety of services and institutions would routinely have to draw on a far wider set of indicators and metrics.

Resistance to expanding the operational definition of safety to include such 'harms' could arise on the grounds that they do not amount to harms at all – perhaps because they are psychological in nature or insufficiently significant. It would seem to be a bad strategy to exclude them simply because they are emotional or psychological in nature, rather than physical: healthcare practice that causes or worsens serious psychological trauma or mental illness is surely unsafe, especially healthcare practice which seeks to manage or alleviate mental illness, just as healthcare which causes or worsens physical injury is unsafe. But it is reasonable to suggest that not all offences or hurts are sufficiently serious to be classified as harms. Much disrespectful speech which treats people as inferior will not actually succeed in making them inferior – because they and others resist and reject the belittling implications – so may not best be seen to actually harm them, if their dignity and social status remain intact.[12] In addition, although unpleasant mental states such as fear, disgust, shame and embarrassment may be perceived as bad, this doesn't mean that people have an interest in not feeling them as such, but only when they are sufficiently serious to actually set back their interests.[13] This would indicate that low-level offences should not always be classified as harms or harmful, at least in the sense normally adopted in patient safety policy. Furthermore, the status of dignitary harms as offensive or injurious is liable to be contested, as the disrespectfulness of a comment or action will be at least partly dependent on the setting, both the specific environment and the more general social and historical context, including cultural norms and expectations and the identity of the recipient and instigator of the act in question. Whether a dignitary harm is in fact harmful will require some understanding of the subjective psychological states of those involved, and the relevant intentions and impact may be disputed. These factors suggest that the status of dignitary harms as harms is, at least sometimes, highly contestable.

It is not at all clear, however, that all dignitary harms fall below the level at which they might be considered salient for patient safety. People's interests may not always be meaningfully set back by minor hurts or insults, but they certainly can be by major ones. In addition, there are circumstances in which cumulative minor offences can cause harms, and sometime qualify as harms. Repeated incidents of disrespectful treatment, as experienced by many racially minoritized, trans and disabled people, for example, while each relatively minor taken on their own can collectively inflict harm over a course of medical care or a lifetime, and acquire contextual significance in ways that also contribute to social injustice. Words or behaviour that could be only negligibly hurtful when directed at one person could be deeply hurtful when directed at another, because of their identity, personal history or (assumed) group membership. And humiliating words or actions from a friend, a mentor, someone otherwise respected or someone who is supposed to be in a caring role may be more damaging than the words of a stranger. This suggests that a lot of contextual information is needed to assess the harmfulness of dignitary harms. While context will also be relevant to identifying and assessing the physical harms that patient safety has traditionally focused on, their harmfulness is less likely to depend on the personal identity, status and history of those involved.

While these considerations may not be conclusive, it should be clear that it is at least reasonable to suggest that some dignitary harms ought to be considered within the scope of safety – and, at the very least, it's contestable whether they are or are not.[14] Operationalizing safety requires, then, a justified decision whether or not to include dignitary harms. The outcome of such a decision will significantly change the scope of safety practice and research, including which services are and are not thought to be safe and why. But operationalizing safety when it includes dignitary harms is liable to be more difficult than operationalizing safety when it only includes physical and major psychological harms. Dignitary harms may be more difficult to conclusively identify because there are liable to be differences in how particular words and actions are interpreted by different people, and the way communicative behaviours are intended may differ from the way they are received. Dignitary harms are, moreover, not always visible or public, and can occur in one-to-one communication or go unnoticed by bystanders. The combination of the highly contextual nature of dignitary harms and their often subtle and contestable nature makes it difficult to come up with a definitive specification of how to identify and measure them.

It is also worth noting that inclusion of dignitary harms within the scope of safety would blur the line between 'safety' as a healthcare concern and other aspects of healthcare quality such as 'person-centredness', 'care', 'respect' and 'equity'. The more typical operationalization of patient safety in terms of physical harm will be much more aligned with quality dimensions such as 'clinical effectiveness' and 'timeliness' – with safety failures contributing to worse clinical outcomes, delayed diagnoses and extended hospital stays or readmissions. But if patient safety concerns also include those relating to dignitary harms, then safety failures will sometimes be directly relevant to assessments of how equitable, caring, responsive and patient-centred services are too.

4.3.2 Harm, risk and safety cultures

We have suggested that the operationalization of patient safety is challenging because what counts as a harm is contested. Our argument now turns to the notion – recognized in the framing of, and many discussions within, the contemporary field of patient safety – that tackling safety depends upon attention not just to harms but to risks of harms, and to the cultures and structures that manage such risks. We suggest that operationalizing risks is an even more uncertain prospect than operationalizing harms.

Consider the following scenario: a patient is having a central line (central venous catheter) inserted for the administration of intravenous antibiotics. Prior to the intervention, the catheter insertion site is not properly cleaned and the medical team do not follow handwashing or equipment-sterilization guidelines. The patient does not develop a central line infection, suffers no harm from the intervention and benefits from the antibiotics. Would it be right to say that the patient has been subject to safe care? Our instinct is that, although the patient has avoided harm, their care has not been safe. They have been exposed to significant risk of harm, because they have been subjected to practices which are liable to cause infection and illness and have been lucky enough to escape it. This suggests that it is not just concrete harms that characterize unsafe care; rather, care is unsafe where the risk of iatrogenic harm is not adequately managed. That is, patient safety as a field of practice must be concerned not just with the actual harm caused by healthcare, but also by its disposition to harm.

It can be quite difficult to pinpoint exactly what is wrong with putting someone at risk of harm when that harm never materializes and the ethics of risk have generally received less attention than the ethics of harm.[15] While it might seem like a rather unlikely analogy, we think that comparing this case with the 'republican' conception of liberty – and, specifically the ideas of 'reliability' and 'resilience' embodied in that conception – helps to illuminate the wrong of risky practices. Liberty is widely understood to be an important political value. The dominant conception of liberty is sometimes called 'negative' liberty and captures the idea that someone is free to the extent that their choices are not interfered with. English philosopher J. S. Mill famously defended the importance of negative liberty, arguing that people should be free to act as they choose, so long as their actions do not harm others or deprive them of their own freedoms.[16] But other philosophers who agree that freedom is an extremely important value argue that the idea of negative freedom does not capture what is so significant about it. Phillip Pettit, one of the most prominent defenders of the so-called republican conception of liberty, argues that liberty is best understood as 'non-domination' rather than freedom from interference.[17]

By way of illustration of republican freedom, consider a community of people who are ruled by a powerful but benevolent despot. As it happens, the despot does not interfere with the activities of her subjects, and they are relatively free to do as they please. She has the power, however, if she wishes to use it, to force them to do whatever she wants. As she is benevolent, she refrains from using this power, and her subjects are therefore free, according to the negative conception of liberty. Pettit, and other republican liberals, think there is something wrong with this account: while the subjects are in fact free from interference, they are subject to the constant possibility of arbitrary interference. Liberty, republican theorists claim, requires not just freedom from actual incidents of interference, but structural protection from interference. Without such protections – provided by measures such as democratic participation and representation, a mixed constitution, the rule of law and so on – people will live in a state of uncertainty, as their liberty will be contingent on their ruler not exercising her power to arbitrarily interfere with their choices and actions.

While patient safety is clearly different from liberty in surface-level respects, there is an important comparison to be drawn. Republican conceptions of freedom emphasize the structural features which ensure (or at least promote) the reliable maintenance of states of liberty, rather than just *de facto* freedom from intervention. Similarly, while avoidance of harm is a crucial part of patient safety, it is not sufficient for healthcare to be deemed safe. If a healthcare organization takes many risks with respect to the safety of patients, by forgoing procedures, protocols and patterns of behaviour which are known to reduce harms, then they create a state of insecurity with respect to safety which can itself be considered unsafe. Safety requires the presence of processes and behaviours that ensure and assure people of the avoidance of harm, not just the avoidance of harm *per se*. One aspect of these conditions may be a visible and explicit commitment to promote safety on the part of an organization and individuals within it, although this will not, of course, be sufficient to ensure safety. While it is impossible to remove all possibilities of poor outcomes from healthcare, such measures create conditions where patients feel, and are, as securely safe as can be reasonably expected, and not just coincidentally or arbitrarily safe. The processes and behaviours in question must, of course, be identified on the basis that they reliably prevent harm but, given such a link has been reasonably secured, upholding the procedures and protocols is itself an important part of securing patient safety as preventing harm. This highlights some important characteristics of safe care: namely, that avoidance of harm is resilient and not arbitrary, that is, that safety is not dependent on good luck, and that care would continue to be safe in alternative possible scenarios.

A wide range of different interventions and protocols are employed for patient safety. These include physical constraints and aids – such as the use of differently shaped terminal probes to prevent using incorrect anaesthetics in surgery, and of sealed, single-use needles and scalpel blades to prevent infection – and formal procedures and protocols – such as a requirement to wear gloves, masks and sanitary clothing in certain environments, hand-washing protocols, mandated use of checklists and the required use of warning lights in doorways to indicate operation of X-ray machinery. Safety procedures also include more open-ended conventions, such as active encouragement for everyone, no matter how junior, to speak up about things that don't seem right and the use of multi-disciplinary team meetings and other opportunities to discuss emerging or potential issues in settings that are not urgent nor at the bedside or point of care. For some of these procedures it is reasonably easy to know whether and when they are in place, but others are more difficult to implement and monitor, because they depend on people not just performing certain observable activities, but also having certain attitudes. The idea of a 'safety culture' is used to describe organizations which are characterized by beliefs, attitudes, behaviours and values that tend to promote and reproduce safe care.[18] This broadly captures the same thing that we are talking about here: the set of 'background' conditions which tend to promote safety.

Defining, operationalizing and measuring a safety culture are all extremely difficult, in part because what is needed to manage the risk of harm will be very different in different contexts and also because safe practice involves a wide array of different activities and attitudes which will act in concert and interact in complex ways. Some behaviours may be relatively causally ineffective on their own, but when taken as part of a set of activities and measures, be an important part of building and maintaining a safe healthcare environment. This suggests that more holistic, evaluative assessments of safety are needed, rather than calculative or additive approaches where the contribution of each component activity is assessed separately and treated as independent. Operationalizing risk is more difficult. While it is more or less easy to identify when a determinate event has happened, it is more difficult to identify when a similar kind of event has been avoided, because counterfactual scenarios can be predicted or hypothesized but not observed. Moreover, in a healthcare environment when risk of harm is very well managed, there will nonetheless, inevitably, be some iatrogenic harms – some infections, for example, are likely to occur even if very careful efforts are taken to avoid them. This suggests another reason why it may be difficult to operationalize and measure a more risk-oriented conception of safety: namely, some harms which are characteristic of unsafe care will be generated by safe care. This means that observing iatrogenic harms, at least individually, will not be a sufficient indicator of unsafe practice. In order to identify safety issues, it will also be necessary to take a broader look at patterns of harm, the plausible causal basis of harms and their reasonable avoidability. Moreover, while there is certainly contestation around the meaning and scope of harm, as discussed in Section 4.3.1, there is liable to be even greater contestation about acceptable risk levels in relation to patient safety. Different people and institutions operate, often justifiably, with different risk–benefit compromises, and this will partly be a matter of social convention and may be impacted by external social, political and economic factors. Added together, all these characteristics make it likely that a risk-based conception of safety will be much more difficult to operationalize than a traditional harm-based conceptualization. It will often not be possible to identify particular acts or cases as 'safe' or 'unsafe' as, on a risk-based conception of safety, this is an assessment that might only be applied to groups of cases, in comparison to relevantly similar cases under different background conditions.

The analogy between liberty and safety may be taken even further without stretching it too thin: inevitably, across a population across time, there will be some undue interference in people's freedom, due, for example, to criminal activity, misapplication of policy and government overreach, and human and system error. A just state will have processes for managing this, such as a fair and well-funded criminal justice system, procedures for checking the implementation of policies and correcting any issues, and a system of compensation for those who have been wrongly interfered with or prevented from enacting their rights. A good state does not throw up its hands when error or injustice has been committed but takes steps to understand and rectify it. This creates a degree of assurance and reassurance in an inevitably imperfect system. Similarly, healthcare will produce iatrogenic harms, and a goal of eliminating these would probably be erroneous in many contexts. While a safe healthcare system may not completely eliminate iatrogenic harms, it will incorporate processes which learn from, respond to, apologize for, mitigate and compensate for iatrogenic harms and risks to patients.

The definition of safety in terms of avoidable iatrogenic harm seems at first glance relatively straightforward. A closer look suggests that this is a far more normatively laden and contested landscape than it first appears, however. Operationalizing safety requires settling normative questions about the appropriate scope of harm and defining and measuring complex and relatively intangible concepts like risk. Depending on how safety is characterized, operationalizing safety may also involve defining and measuring concepts like disrespect, which are normative, highly interpretive and have a subjective component.

4.4 Quality by numbers and the logic of improvement

To recap, the way that efficiency and safety have typically been conceived in contexts where healthcare quality is being schematically defined and specified emphasizes relatively 'hard' factors. Efficiency is often operationalized in terms of a restricted set of institutional inputs – such as money, time, equipment and workforce – and outputs – such as completed procedures and staff utilization. Safety is often operationalized in terms of (avoidance of) a specified set of relatively discrete bad events and outcomes. We have argued that these emphases are not inherent to these quality dimensions but represent a particular approach to characterizing and constructing knowledge claims in these domains. There are other currents within healthcare improvement research and practice that would resist the construction of these dimensions as 'objective' and 'hard', and also contexts where the imperative of demonstrating measurable changes in these dimensions moves somewhat into the background (e.g. where improvement activities and emphases switch to longer-term and broader considerations, as discussed in Chapter 7). Nonetheless, the emphasis on hardness remains prominent because most institutionalized approaches to quality place measurability centre-stage.

The attractiveness of 'harder' characterizations of quality is not difficult to understand. Such characterizations, in principle at least, enable relatively clear-cut answers to questions about healthcare quality and give unambiguous directions for improvement. If safety is thought of as the absence of a range of unequivocally bad events, then it is relatively easy to say whether things have improved by counting the occurrence of these bad events over time. But if, as we have suggested, safety is understood to be a more holistic phenomenon it will be much more difficult to conclusively measure improvements. We have also shown that making assessments of efficiency always involves making trade-offs between different resources and ends, so there will always be interpretation and judgement involved. Only considering a limited set of resources and ends radically constrains the factors feeding into judgements about efficiency and its improvement, and makes it much easier to make such assessments confidently. Using standardized or established measures and data sources in order to evidence claims about efficiency is liable to make assessments even less contested and allows for comparisons to be made over time and across settings. By contrast, acknowledging the wider set of resources and range of ends, and the ways that these are conceptualized and prioritized from the perspectives of different vantage points, stakeholders and actors, makes assessments of efficiency much more complicated. This is because the latter requires us to ask *for whom* and *to what end* changes are efficient. Adopting a harder characterization of certain quality dimensions makes pragmatic sense in light of the broad practical motivation to operationalize quality in improvement work: when measuring something complex and vague, it is good to have a blueprint which defines and characterizes it more concretely. The danger is that operationalization is taken to signal not just the beginning of positive action but also (problematically) the end of any need for reflection. For example, settling on an operational definition and set of measures might be taken as the endpoint of a process of considering various different framings of a concept, beyond which it no longer seems necessary or even possible to question the appropriateness of the one adopted.

The process of operationalizing healthcare quality also, we argue, reflects an underlying 'logic of improvement'. As we discussed in the previous chapter, the idea of healthcare quality has come to reflect a schematic way of thinking about healthcare and its improvement. That is, it represents an approach to determining how good instances of healthcare are which proceeds by developing specifications of good healthcare against which to measure and predict actual practice. This approach is schematic, insofar as it involves drawing up quality schema, which explicitly set out what good practice looks like before seeking to measure and understand how good particular services and systems are. It is also reductive, insofar as it breaks down the idea of good healthcare and its dimensions into more easily manageable components. It is, therefore, unsurprising that such an approach emphasizes aspects of healthcare and indicators of good and bad healthcare practice that can be clearly and simply described and measured – that is, that it tends to produce and value harder versions of concepts. This schematic approach to understanding quality not only explains why harder versions of dimensions such as safety feature in improvement discourses and practices but arguably helps shed light on the central place given to more-easily-operationalizable dimensions of quality. There are good substantive grounds for the prominence given to effectiveness, efficiency and safety in discussions of healthcare quality, but this prominence is likely reinforced because they are relatively amenable to schematic thinking.

Because of the reductive tendencies of such schematization, operationalization can go hand-in-hand with decision-making which, in practice, avoids confronting ethical issues or, at least, renders ethical issues into a disguised form. That is, it can present questions of quality and improvement as more or less black and white issues – merely requiring understanding of whether a service conforms to a specific quality schema – rather than seeing operationalized quality concepts as pragmatic representations of a much more complex and contested underlying reality. When operationalization is not preceded by ethical deliberation, it will reflect implicit assumptions about the best way to conceptualize particular quality concepts. But, even if it is preceded by ethical reflection, operationalization can nonetheless obscure ethical tensions once operational definitions exist as tools which are used in practice to make changes to systems and evaluative claims about them.

It is not, we suggest, so much that some dimensions of quality are 'hard' by their nature, but that they have been 'hardened' – that is, characterized in more measurable, countable and simplified ways, which makes them more manageable as quality improvement subjects and goals. The examples we have developed and discussed in this chapter suggest that lying behind these useful simplifications there is considerable space for disagreement about *how* to operationalize safety and efficiency, which is underpinned by differing accounts of the functions and desired outcomes of healthcare and of what should be prioritized. Many valued aspects of healthcare are difficult to measure definitively – even within these putatively hard dimensions of quality. So claims about quality that are based on formal measurement are unlikely to reflect everything that matters. This makes it difficult to say with certainty what better and worse practice and outcomes look like. In addition, even when it is possible to measure valued characteristics of healthcare, this will not necessarily generate determinate claims about quality and improvement, and even when there is agreement about what matters in healthcare, delivering good healthcare and healthcare improvements involves balancing and optimizing the different things that matter. Our examination of efficiency indicates that it is necessary to balance and trade off valued ends in order to make claims about efficient functioning – even with agreement about the relevant costs and benefits and knowledge of their magnitude. The characterization of quality and quality dimensions in discrete, measurable terms supports a 'maximizing' logic of quality and improvement, where valued healthcare goods are prespecified and healthcare services and systems are deemed better insofar as they have more of them (or less of prespecified 'bads'). This somewhat misleadingly enables improvers to focus on maximizing simplified 'outputs' rather than having to think about complex clusters of relevant values and how they might be jointly considered and balanced together.

While we recognize the pragmatic value of simplified assessments of better and worse healthcare and broadly 'maximizing' thinking, we also caution that it comes with real dangers, including of encouraging improvers to overlook and undervalue things and people that matter, and to produce simplistic improvement narratives. Some of the more contested aspects of efficiency and safety are difficult to measure because they are contextual and depend upon people's subjective states, like disrespect and humiliation, or because they are not readily accessible from an institutional perspective and may have an impact on institutions only through their indirect effects, like staff well-being and satisfaction. This chapter has highlighted how orthodox operationalizations of efficiency and safety can reflect narrow institutional perspectives, which do not necessarily reflect either the broader social values that healthcare might aim to promote – such as well-being and relational equality – or the personal needs and interests of the people who work in and are served by those institutions. Operational constructions of quality dimensions embody ethically relevant standpoints. So the way that desirable and undesirable features and outcomes of healthcare are characterized can implicitly or explicitly value or devalue, acknowledge or overlook, particular people and groups. Recognizing this wider context of claims about healthcare quality and its dimensions shows those claims to be much more defeasible and partial, as it highlights their limited scope and perspective. Appreciating these limitations is essential if operational claims are to be used with wisdom and restraint. And acknowledging the things that matter outside of operational definitions has the potential to enrich an understanding of what healthcare systems can and should look like.

The 'maximizing' tendencies of schematic representations and operationalization of quality and quality dimensions – and the linked treatment of different quality dimensions as largely discrete phenomena – also have the potential to obscure some of the tensions between different dimensions of quality that we highlighted in Chapter 3. When safety and efficiency are treated as modular, and thus as able to be measured and improved independently, there is a danger of overlooking the ways that changes in some areas of healthcare can change or limit other areas of practice. Sometimes this is just a matter of the opportunity costs of decisions in a resource-limited context. But sometimes different dimensions of quality can conceptually overlap and come into tension with one another, as when improving safety by increasing the resilience and adaptability of systems means that far more slack is built into the system than might be deemed 'efficient' – for example, when burnout and errors are reduced by increasing the size of the workforce or restricting their workload. Taking a more holistic view of quality and reflecting on how schematic representations of quality relate to broader ideas of good healthcare will sometimes involve challenging a maximalist logic and thinking about how different healthcare functions and values fit together – and when they might come into tension. Emphasizing the practical and normative decisions that are involved in operationalizing dimensions of quality, even those which appear relatively hard at first glance, can help to demonstrate that such tensions are not so much a problem as an inevitable feature of any attempts to measure and improve complex human systems which are multi-functional and operate with a variety of valued ends.

When quality concepts are rendered into hard formulations, they can come to be synonymous with worrying about particular kinds of mistake. Inefficiency, as we have illustrated, can simply be conceptualized in terms of financial waste or mismanagement of staff time. Unsafe care can simply be described in relation to major physical harms which occur in healthcare. Quality improvement, in relation to efficiency and safety, is therefore taken to require rectification, and ideally elimination, of these issues. These characterizations prioritize the operationalizability of these quality concepts, emphasizing features of care that are relatively easy to identify and measure, hence giving the impression of hardness. Such hardness can be self-reinforcing because of the high value placed on quantitative evidence.

In this chapter, we have argued that 'hard' conceptualizations of quality concepts mask much more contested and evaluative conceptual and moral realities. There are other ways of thinking about these important concepts which, though perhaps more difficult to definitively schematize and measure, capture something significant about their nature and value. We have highlighted, in particular, how consideration of personal resources and ends, and the way these feed into and intersect with institutional resources and ends, affect assessments of efficiency, and how defining and looking beyond conventional conceptions of biomedical harm have the potential to change assessments of safety. We have argued that operationalization of quality concepts involves the assertion of relatively definite boundaries of what is in and out of the specification. This is valuable, and sometimes necessary, for the practical implementation of many quality and improvement activities. But it can make it difficult to deal with uncertainty and vague boundaries and gives a misleading impression of definiteness. Using hard, circumscribed operational definitions enables those involved in healthcare quality and improvement activities to make strong claims that some instance of care or care system is 'efficient' or 'safe', but this can paper over all sorts of mistakes and issues which don't come under the formal definitions being deployed. Care can be efficient or safe in key, prespecified respects, while at the same time not doing justice to other important but less easily operationalizable aspects of efficiency and safety. One upshot of this is that what officially counts as good quality care and how patients and staff experience and evaluate care might come apart quite substantially.

5 THE 'SOFTNESS' OF QUALITY

Some dimensions of healthcare quality unmistakably reflect and promote particular social and interpersonal values. When someone says that healthcare should be equitable, person-centred, respectful, caring and so on, they pick out attributes that point to and validate certain social attitudes and conventions. Such dimensions have a relatively evident normative character, that is, they are obviously evaluative and readily prompt ethical questions about their meaning and implications. By comparison, dimensions such as safety, efficiency and effectiveness, discussed in the previous chapter, are also normative in character but this normativity can be obscured under a veil of objectivity or hardness. Defining and assessing 'softer' dimensions of healthcare quality are more obviously likely to also involve attention to 'subjective' considerations – such as people's mental states and perspectives, and their related social identities and positions – and appeal to more open-ended descriptive and qualitative characterizations. Such open-endedness and subjectivity have the potential to generate disagreement. Whether an instance of care is 'respectful', for example, is liable to be contestable, not only because the broader meaning and scope of 'respect' are open to interpretation and subject to contextual variation but also because different people might reasonably have different interpretations of what happened in a particular care encounter, including the intention, meaning and implications of words and actions.

This generates a puzzle – how can improvers ask of healthcare systems and services that they be equitable and just, and deliver care that is person-centred, respectful, dignified, caring and so on, if they don't have a clear idea of what these values mean and what they look like in practice? Indeed, if, as we argued in Chapter 4, defining and measuring dimensions of healthcare quality that initially appear more objective also involve making value judgements, then this puzzle extends even further. How can healthcare quality be practically assessed and improved if the meaning and nature of quality are indeterminate and reflect people's diverse values and purposes as much as any 'external' or 'mind-independent' reality?

In this chapter we explore how it might be possible to avoid practical inertia while, at the same time, acknowledging the open-endedness of healthcare quality assessments. We approach this challenge by looking in more detail at the concepts of equality and person-centredness, which are commonly invoked in quality discourses but subject to substantial indeterminacy and disagreement. As with efficiency and safety in the previous chapter, we are partly interested in discussing these concepts in their own right – considering what range of things improvers have in mind when they cite them as aspects of healthcare quality. But we are also interested in them because they help to illustrate, and amplify, our account of the slipperiness of appeals to quality. The chapter therefore continues the argument, begun in Chapter 3, for a pluralistic and pragmatic conception of healthcare quality. In particular, it investigates what underpins the limits of operationalization (the theme of the previous chapter) and makes a case for positively embracing open-endedness and variation in the way improvers understand and use quality concepts. It thereby highlights the need for healthcare improvement to encompass an interpretive and dialogical culture alongside a scientific one. In short, the chapter pulls together and underlines our case for emphasizing the underlying 'softness' of quality, in contrast to the hard image conveyed by the influence of schematic thinking.

5.1 Disagreement and variation in quality dimensions

Disagreement about the meaning of healthcare concepts, including quality concepts, can be substantial and intractable. Sometimes disagreement is overt, when different research teams, institutions and official bodies develop and use different, inconsistent definitions of quality dimensions. In Chapters 3 and 4, we highlighted several examples of this phenomenon, including variation in the high-level definition of quality dimensions and differences in their operationalization and specification. Such inconsistent definitions can obviously lead to different assessments of quality dimensions such as safety or effectiveness. But sometimes disagreement about the meaning of dimensions is more implicit. A healthcare practitioner or organization may claim that care is 'safe' or 'effective' and attribute this to an increase or decrease in a limited set of variables or an assessment according to a particular benchmark. If two healthcare organizations characterize themselves as 'safe', but each uses a different tool for measuring and assessing patient safety, then there can be said to be an implicit conflict in the definition of safety, even if the differences are not in fact brought to light. In this section, we look beyond these more straightforward examples of explicit or implicit disagreement, and we summarize three features of quality concepts that help produce high levels of variation and contestation – their being open to interpretation, their contextual variability and their subjectivity.

5.1.1 Openness to interpretation

First, as the last two chapters have underlined, quality concepts are open to interpretation. That is, their definition or meaning leaves space for different, and potentially inconsistent, understandings of what they require in practice. The words used to label some dimensions of healthcare quality are used extensively in non-technical ways outside of healthcare contexts. Equality, timeliness, efficiency and safety are all good examples of this. In healthcare policy and practice, a commitment to a healthcare value like 'equality' or 'timeliness', or a claim that a service or system embodies (or fails to embody) one of these concepts, can be variously interpreted because these are relatively loose, evaluative, concepts, that are used in a range of ways. The broadness and widespread applicability of quality concepts are arguably central to their plausibility and perceived significance as guiding healthcare values – part of what makes them important as healthcare values is their importance as social values more widely. But this same breadth creates challenges when improvement activities are assumed to depend on the use of operationalized concepts. The gap between the widespread social salience of concepts and the demands of making them 'usable' in specific practices seems greatest in the case of conspicuously 'soft' concepts – those concepts that are strikingly, and perhaps inherently, interpretative in nature. We illustrate this with the concept of 'equality' and other quality concepts associated with it.

When a claim is made that a health service is, or should be, equitable or egalitarian, this can mean a wide range of things. Appeals to the value of equality simply do not make practical sense if they are interpreted as calling for equality in every possible respect. To make sense they must rest on an implicit or explicit claim about what or who should be equal and in what respects. When thinking about equality in the context of health and healthcare, improvers might be interested in how health-related *resources* are distributed, for example, how much money is given to health services in different areas of the country per capita, or what level of health resources, including workforce, buildings and equipment, are available to different services. Or they might be concerned with the *opportunities* individuals have to access and receive healthcare, which might include considerations of geographic accessibility; opening times; physical, telephonic and digital care opportunities; language and translation; as well as the provision of funding for healthcare services and professionals. Inequalities in these areas might be thought to be problematic either in themselves or because of their consequences, for example, on health or other aspects of personal or social well-being. If improvers are interested in how health and healthcare *outcomes* are distributed across individuals, groups and populations, these can be conceptualized in different ways. For example, analysis might focus on the major clinical incidents and shorter-term biomedical markers or functional assessments that are often measured as healthcare outcomes, or might also or instead look at longer term and more diffuse consequences, including experiences of health or well-being and satisfaction with care. Such inequalities might be thought to be unfair themselves (inequitable) or to lead to further unfairness insofar as they limit opportunities.

Improvers might also, or ultimately, be interested in how resources, opportunities and outcomes are systematically associated with patterns of social disadvantage that reveal deeper inequalities and differences in status.[1] This more *relational* emphasis might justify a focus on questions of who is included in the design and arrangement of healthcare services; how trust in institutions can sustain relationships of mutual respect; and how health opportunities and outcomes link to broader social issues and access to other social and personal goods. Equality can be interpreted, then, in a dizzying range of ways – indeed, almost any political or ethical position can be redescribed in terms of some kind of equality, whether it's equal rights, equal resources, equal outcomes, equal opportunities, equal status, equal power and so on. This ubiquity and shape-shifting to reflect different political and ethical concerns highlight both the significance of equality as a moral concept and its weakness as a goal or commitment. Claims that a change has improved the equality of a healthcare system, or claims that a service is 'equitable' or 'inequitable', can appear to be expressing something morally noteworthy, while at the same time remaining largely devoid of content insofar as the kind of equality or equity in question remains unspecified.

The wide recognition of a concept's value combined with varied usage may mean that while there is agreement about its significance when it is invoked in relatively vague and general terms, there is less agreement about more specific definitions. In the previous two chapters we discussed in some depth how operational definitions close down the range of interpretability of quality concepts. On the one hand, specification work can facilitate agreement on what to do or say in practice. But, on the other hand, a more specific definition can end up focusing on just some aspects of the valued entity and missing out others, thus opening up a gap between the adopted technical definition of the concept and a broader sense of its meaning. This may result in charges that while a service is claimed to be egalitarian because it meets a specific, technical definition of equality, it is in fact problematically unequal in some important respects. While a concept's being open to interpretation leaves space for misunderstanding and disagreement to arise, closing down its definition via operationalization does nothing to resolve disagreements but merely finds a stipulative way forward for limited purposes.

5.1.2 Contextual variation

Second, quality concepts can be subject to contextual and cultural variation. It can be appropriate to use different definitions of a particular concept in different contexts or in relation to different population groups. The range of intelligible variation may be greater for some concepts than others but there is reason to suppose that many healthcare values are subject to significant contextual variation. Contextual variation need not amount to disagreement about the meaning of a quality concept, as the scope of application for different definitions or characterizations may not overlap. If different conceptualizations of a given concept apply only in distinct settings, there will be no conflict between apparently inconsistent definitions. But where there is contextual variation in the meaning attached to a concept a certain amount of interpretive work is needed to understand what the appropriate or correct characterization of it is, given the context and environmental characteristics in question. Care must be taken, for example, to ensure that definitions are used only in contexts where they are appropriate.

Whether an instance of care is 'person-centred', for example, may be understood quite differently in different settings. Person-centredness broadly captures the ideas that healthcare treats patients as persons, rather than seeing them just in terms of their pathology or symptoms, and centres healthcare around patients rather than institutional or clinical interests and aims. Many of the definitions of person-centred care that have been developed are intended to be generic, overarching definitions of person-centredness that do not specify a particular healthcare setting or patient group.[2] Other definitions have been developed for specific settings, including rehabilitation,[3] nursing,[4] dementia care,[5] primary care[6] and mental healthcare.[7] Insofar as these differ in their scope of application, they can be understood to be not strictly conflicting but rather parallel and limited in their appropriate usage. A patchwork of definitions has the potential to enable highly nuanced assessments of person-centred care, but it also limits the generalizability and comparability of claims and assessments of person-centredness.

Definitional variation that has the potential to be more problematic can arise between generic and context-specific definitions of person-centredness, and between different generic definitions. If a generic definition of person-centred care is substantively different from a context-specific definition in its particular dimensions or emphases, how should one definition be chosen as more appropriate? It is possible to compare, for example, an influential generic definition of person-centredness with an influential rehabilitation-specific definition (see Table 2). Both definitions in principle include rehabilitation care contexts within their scope. But while there is certainly overlap between them, the generic definition includes emphases not mentioned in the rehabilitation-specific definition, such as coordination of care and involvement of family and friends. Should this be taken to imply that these aspects of person-centred care, while widely applicable, are not in fact applicable in the case of rehabilitation, or less important and so not to be treated as key aspects? Is such divergence unremarkable and unproblematic or does the divergence flag up a problem with one or both definitions – that they

Table 2 A More Generic and a More Specific Definition of Person-Centred Care

More generic (Gerteis et al. 1993)	More specific – to rehabilitation (Leplege et al. 2007)
Seven primary dimensions of patient-centred care:	Four main interpretations of person-centredness:
1. Respect for patients' values, preferences and expressed needs	1. Addressing the person's specific and holistic properties
2. Coordination and integration of care	2. Addressing the person's difficulties in everyday life
3. Information, communication and education	3. The person as expert: participation and empowerment
4. Physical comfort	4. Respect the person 'behind' the impairment or the disease
5. Emotional support and alleviation of fear and anxiety	
6. Involvement of family and friends	
7. Transition and continuity	

Source: Gerteis et al. (1993) pp5–12; Leplege et al. (2007).

either miss out some key aspects of person-centred rehabilitation care or include some unnecessary components in their characterization of it? There is no uncontentious way to settle these questions.

Contextual variation in the use of quality concepts may, then, sometimes be largely unproblematic, because there is little or no overlap between different core contexts to which different quality definitions apply. But sometimes it will be challenging, and may require careful deliberation, to determine which of several possible definitions is most useful for a particular context and purpose, where this will require attention not just to the care setting but also the reasons for which care quality is being assessed. One upshot of such contextual variation is that it may not be possible to meaningfully compare evidence about what appears to be the same concept across settings, if substantially different definitions are in use.

5.1.3 Subjectivity

Third, the meaning and application of some quality concepts are, at least in part, subjective. This means that considerations such as what comes within its scope, whether the object of consideration is present and to what extent, and whether some activities promote or endorse it, are in part dependent on the experiential perspectives (including situational interpretations and psychological experiences) of particular individuals. Subjective experience is also influenced by cultural variations across time and space that reflect the systems of meanings, norms and expected social relations that help constitute subjectivity.

Person-centredness is a key quality concept that clearly illustrates the relevance of subjectivity. Determining what features care must have to be called person-centred and whether some instance of care or a service is in fact person-centred both depend to some extent on the subjective experiences of individuals. Depending on the capacities, preferences and characteristics of individual patients, person-centred care may require more or less support in decision-making, a greater or lesser emphasis on involvement and participation, and different approaches to communication and relationship-building. More broadly, assuming that person-centred care requires consideration of the preferences, interests and values of patients and their families, it will have different implications for different people. For example, in making efforts to build a strong patient-clinician relationship, and to support open communication, determining whether an instance of care is person-centred will likely require some consideration of the subjective experiences of the individual patients, family members and clinicians, as it is difficult to make an objective or externally observed assessment of these characteristics. Of course, there may be ways of assessing these features that don't involve measuring the subjective experience of those involved – by considering whether care planning and decision-making tools were used, for example, or via observation of consultations by communication experts. But these capture only part of these features of person-centredness, and consideration of subjective experiences will at very least comprise distinctive and relevant input into assessments of person-centredness.

If different patients experience similar care scenarios very differently – because of their distinctive individual needs or values and/or because of differences in cultural expectations – this won't necessarily amount to disagreement about what is person-centred in a broader sense, if the individual experience of patients is a key part of understanding person-centred care. But it does indicate that knowing whether a particular instance of care is person-centred may require a good deal of very specific contextual information, including subjective assessments, and may not be exhausted by knowing that it has certain generic, observable features.

Other healthcare values associated with quality also include some subjective elements, at least under many interpretations. Returning to equality, more relational as opposed to more distributive characterizations – those which emphasize respect, dignity and relationships characterized by mutuality and trust – more obviously have subjective components. While there are some instances of disrespect and inegalitarian attitudes that are relatively clear-cut and would be widely recognized as such by casual observers, often the facts of whether someone is treated as equal or accorded equal status, and whether they are shown appropriate respect, will require understanding of the subjective attitudes and experiences of the person involved. Disrespectful treatment can manifest via microaggressions or words and actions that would have been unremarkable if aimed at a different person – someone who is not a member of a minoritized group or without certain personal characteristics, for example. This means that understanding whether some action, process or system is relationally inegalitarian is liable to require a good deal of contextual understanding and interpretation, including understanding the intentions, attitudes and social positions and identities of those involved.

When we talk about quality concepts being open to interpretation, contextually variable and subjective we are, importantly, not suggesting that their definition and interpretation are entirely indeterminate and up-for-grabs. But these three features do indicate a high degree of open-endedness and flexibility in assessing and evaluating healthcare quality. Once again, these features do not necessarily imply *disagreement* about the definition of quality dimensions. The different conceptualizations of dimensions that are invoked in different contexts may diverge but will only contradict one another insofar as their domains of application overlap and they generate incompatible accounts of what would be 'good' and 'better' in any given care context. It is certainly the case, however, that, in general, divergent operational definitions of concepts such as person-centredness and equality might quite reasonably be applied to the same case. In principle, this means that an instance of care, or an improvement intervention, could be described in ways that are, at least on the surface, contradictory – as both egalitarian and inegalitarian, or as making things more person-centred and less person-centred. Similarly, when a degree of subjectivity is built into the definition of a quality dimension, then different subjective interpretations will not necessarily amount to disagreement about its meaning but may instead suggest that its manifestation in practice will take different forms. These phenomena necessitate careful reflection on the meaningful comparability of quality claims across contexts, as in many cases they indicate that frameworks and assessments of quality will not be widely generalizable. The open-endedness and variability of some 'soft' quality concepts pose a conundrum for improvers. How far should they try to 'pin down' these concepts to give them a more consistent and firmer shape? Or how far should they embrace, or at least look for ways to live with, this open-endedness? This is the ground we will explore in the remainder of the chapter. We suggest that there is value in looking in both these directions, but we highlight particularly the positive case for embracing open-endedness and variability in characterizations of quality.

5.2 Measurement as interpretation

Questions about improvement are often answered by providing higher or lower measurement scores. But how can concepts such as person-centredness and equality be treated as definable, measurable, improvable dimensions of healthcare given (a) the difficulty of pinning them down and (b) the value of contextual variation and relatively open-ended definitions that admit of subjective variation in practice? The highly contested nature and subjective components of values such as equality and person-centredness make it even less obvious that improvers can adequately capture and score them adequately via metrics compared to other, harder concepts. The conceptual richness and multifaceted nature of these concepts make any quantitative measures liable to capture a small part of their value and substance, whereas qualitative measures limit the scope for systematic comparison. In addition, the personal and subjective or inter-subjective nature of person-centredness and aspects of equality means that measures are only likely to capture partial measures or proxies, due to the difficulties of measuring subjective states. Here we explore and discuss these challenges.

It is difficult to capture the conceptual richness of softer quality concepts in quantitative metrics for reasons that will be familiar from the previous two chapters. First, while individual metrics will record some objects and phenomena of relevance to quality measures, they will necessarily present a limited picture. Consider an attempt to measure equity of access to primary care in a geographical region by ethnicity. First, the investigators will need to understand the differential access to primary care services by members of different ethnic groups. This will involve making choices about what to measure and how, including how ethnic groups are characterized and distinguished and how they are measured (by self-identification, for example, or variables such as country of birth, nationality, language spoken at home, skin colour, parents' nationality or country of birth, or religion). Contestation over the meaning of 'ethnicity' and the appropriate ways of distinguishing between different ethnicities, including whether to use and how to construct standardized classifications of ethnicity, mean that there is unlikely to be a single obvious metric, though there may be strong national, institutional or social conventions. Choices will also have to be made as to how to measure access to primary care, including whether to look at primary care as a whole or to separate it out into different services, whether to measure appointment bookings or actual attendance, whether to measure intervention and referral rates or just the fact that an appointment has taken place. Finally, choices will have to be made about how to measure the geographical region: whether to measure equitable access at a regional, sub-regional or institutional level, for example, and whether to measure access by people living within the region (who might access primary care services outside of it) or access to institutions within the region (which might include access by patients living elsewhere). Such decisions will depend on the purposes of measuring equitable access to primary care and which institutions are involved in making and using assessments.

Even once all these questions have been settled, mere difference in levels of access across ethnic groups will unlikely answer questions about *equitable access*; metrics to reflect what levels of access are fair or deserved are also required. If fair access is taken to mean, for example, access according to need, some measure of healthcare need in different ethnic groups will be required. Again, choices will have to be made about how best to conceptualize and measure need, whether, for example, to focus on general measures such as life expectancy and disability-free life expectancy or to consider incidence of diseases and conditions, age of onset, severity, comorbidities and so on, and how far to take into account existing or historical levels of unmet need in different communities. There are, furthermore, many ways of conceptualizing and operationalizing these different interpretations and aspects of need. For each metric employed non-trivial decisions will be made about what data sources to use and how to assess their validity and reliability, how to check and clean data, and how to define variables and exclusions in analysis. When we describe these decisions as 'non-trivial', we mean that they have the potential to make a difference to the analyses and assessments made, but also that they require reasoning and reflection. There may be good reason to choose differently, depending on the broader social and institutional context of measurement and evaluation.

Reviewing the assortment of decisions facing any investigator operationalizing a soft quality concept for measurement illuminates the many paths not taken – the alternative ways of constructing operational definitions and measures that were passed up in favour of others. In other words, it highlights the inherently interpretive nature of measurement processes. Even when the options chosen are well justified and appropriate, they reflect just one way of characterizing that dimension of quality. In the example given, a final set of metrics will reflect not just one way among many of measuring equity, but also one approach to measuring equity of access, one approach to measuring need, one approach to measuring ethnicity and so on.

The matter of measuring quality dimensions is further complicated by the multidimensional and 'fractal' nature of quality concepts. As already highlighted, not only is quality multidimensional but so too are 'single' dimensions of quality. Person-centredness, for example, is understood by many to be multidimensional.[8] In operationalizing and measuring a multidimensional concept, not only must metrics be identified and characterized for each dimension, but the relationship between them must also be characterized. For example, are the metrics for each dimension to remain separate or is there a process for calculating a summary score that weights and combines them? If there is a summary score, are all of the dimensions weighted equally or are some more critical than others in making an overall assessment? Is the summary score an additive or multiplicative function of the dimension scores, or does it involve a holistic, evaluative judgement? Different ways of conceptualizing the relationship between the dimensions will differently characterize the relative importance of different dimensions, the significance of a particular service or instance of care performing well or badly on more than one dimension, and the way that the dimensions interact with one another. If it is deemed inappropriate to generate a summary score from the different metrics of the quality dimension in question, then assessments may be limited in their comparability in practice. In such a scenario, one instance of person-centred care, for example, will only be able to be conclusively and uncontroversially characterized as better than another if it 'dominates' the latter: that is, if it is no worse on any dimensions and better on one or more. If it is worse on any dimensions, its characterization as better will be contestable, even if it is better on all others. Comparisons that use evaluative judgements about the relative merits of different, non-dominating, multidimensional assessments will be normative and contestable.

The fractal quality of this process of operationalization, where each decision about how to characterize a given concept throws up more decisions, must be seen against a background context where different people and teams in comparable positions make different choices, reflecting their explicit or implicit purposes, values and priorities. This range of characterizations reflects the richness of these concepts and highlights how a particular operational definition and set of quantitative metrics captures only part of the meaning and value of quality concepts. While this conceptual richness may be particularly striking in relation to soft quality concepts, particularly if they also capture more quotidian social values, the previous chapter suggested that a similar phenomenon applies to harder quality concepts. Harder and softer quality concepts alike are subject to contextual variation and interpretability – the challenge we are analysing here applies in large measure across the whole set of quality concepts. In addition, in nearly all cases improvers are interested in changes (for better or worse) across the multiple dimensions of quality. Therefore, even if it were only some aspects of quality that were relatively indeterminate, this would still pose the same obstacles to assessing healthcare quality in definitive ways.

One of the reasons why some quality dimensions might be thought to exemplify softness is that they reflect more qualitative phenomena and this poses conspicuous challenges to measurement. Understanding when and to what extent these dimensions have been fulfilled cannot be fully captured by any set of quantitative metrics, and requires a qualitative assessment of the objects in question. This might involve asking people who have knowledge of the service to think and talk or write about their experience of it and asking them to make evaluative judgements of what it is like. Such accounts and judgements can constitute a form of evidence but will not be wholly exhausted by measurable quantities. Whereas the 'harder' concepts discussed in the previous chapter are typically used in ways that disguise their interpretive and evaluative character, the concepts we have discussed in this chapter make this character easy to see and difficult to disguise.

While qualitative evidence is not understood by everyone to be a form of measurement per se, it nonetheless provides information about systems and services that is relevant to quality claims, so – at least in theory – it can play a comparable role to quantitative measurement in healthcare improvement. High levels of interpretation are, however, involved in understanding what qualitative evidence implies about more abstract and summative claims about the quality of healthcare services and instances of care, so qualitative evidence may appear to be less conclusive and more open to disagreement than quantitative evidence. Of course, to reiterate, the apparently definitive quality assessments generated by quantitative evidence help to obscure a great many underpinning value judgements and interpretative decisions, whereas qualitative evidence wears its interpretability on its sleeve. But qualitative evidence tends to operate with smaller sample sizes and qualitative research is less easy to repeat and replicate than quantitative research, due to its comparative open-endedness and highly contextual nature. This means that any assessments made on the basis of it are likely to be fairly qualified and not directly transferable to other contexts without evidence of relevant similarity.

As well as high levels of interpretability, some quality concepts are more likely to have subjective or inter-subjective aspects. As just discussed, whether some instance of care is person-centred is going to depend, at least in part, on the experiences of key individuals involved. Measuring these in such a way that they can be understood by those other than the person experiencing them requires forms of mediation. This might involve putting the experiences and psychological states into words, answering structured questions about experiences and feelings, or perhaps measuring electrical impulses within the brain. Even when the measurement of subjective states is by direct report – asking someone how involved they felt in their care, or whether they are satisfied with a particular service or experience, for example – what is measured is a proxy or mediated representation of the subjective experiences or states themselves. Proxy measures can be reliable indicators of the states they represent, but gaps can also open up between the proxy measure and the objects it is supposed to be representing. For example, if the design of a survey or order of questions systematically affects the answers given by respondents, or if respondents' interpretations of questions and response options differ from those assumed by researchers, then the survey may be measuring something other than what it is claimed to be measuring.[9] Although people can, in theory, misreport their subjective experiences, what we are highlighting here is not straightforwardly an instance of this, and instead a product of the framing effects of questions and survey scenarios, such that findings reflect something about how people respond to the way questions are asked, and not only the experiences or psychological states of interest. While there are valid and reliable ways of measuring subjective experience, using well-designed and tested surveys and techniques, they often measure quite specific aspects of experience or affect, and there are differences between how different surveys measure these phenomena.[10] Broader claims about subjective psychological states such as how satisfied someone was with an experience or the effect of some event or intervention on their well-being must therefore be made with caution.

The kinds of conceptual disagreement, variation, subjectivity and vagueness that we have outlined seem, at first glance, to present a problem. Mainstream healthcare improvement approaches often require the objects of improvements to be assessed by valid and reliable measurement. And it might seem obvious that in order to measure something, and to tell whether it has improved or not, improvers need to be clear what it is that they are measuring. Many who seek to define equality and person-centredness for the purpose of measurement and improvement certainly think so, claiming, for example, that settling on a more precise definition of equity in health is important 'to guide measurement and, hence, accountability' and has practical consequences for 'both policies and measurement'.[11] Others worry that the lack of a 'clear definition and method of measurement' for concepts like person-centredness hampers the implementation of person-centred care.[12] This suggests that disagreement and uncertainty about what is being measured may have to be settled before these important but broad normative concepts can be used for practical improvement purposes.

In the next section, however, we will argue that trying to define such complex normative concepts once and for all and trying to settle on a single model or measure of them is liable to eclipse much of their nuance and richness. Part of what makes concepts such as equality and person-centredness so ethically significant, and makes them important guiding values and aims in healthcare, we will suggest, is precisely their open-endedness. We therefore resist the idea that disagreement must be settled before definitions and measures of softer quality concepts can be used for improvement purposes.

5.3 Embracing open-endedness

Should improvers even seek a shared definition or measure of a quality concept? It is, first, important to acknowledge why they might. Seeking a 'best definition' for concepts could certainly provide practical, local value, helping to justify evidence-informed claims about improvements and good practice. In addition, the value of agreeing shared definitions and metrics stems from the value of coordinated action. That is, with a single definition of an aspect of healthcare quality, diverse healthcare actors and institutions can work towards common goals and make (and compare) measurable improvements in relation to them. When different institutions and teams are using different definitions and metrics, the extent to which improvements are being made can remain unclear and different parts of the overall system can end up pursuing inconsistent goals. The problem of inconsistency is one reason for wanting to pin down the best definition and metric.

Calls to identify the 'best' or 'correct' definition or metric can also stem from claims about the relative truth, validity and appropriateness of the conceptual content of some or one definition or metric over others. Attempts to settle the correct definition and metric of quality concepts might, for example, use philosophical and conceptual analysis or empirical methods like surveys, observation and factor analysis to argue the case for one definition over others. These arguments can be deployed in different ways: they might be used to make epistemically realist claims – that is, about the 'true' definition of the quality concept of interest, whether in general or for a particular care context. Or they might be used more pragmatically, to indicate why one definition or metric is liable to be better or more useful than others given a particular set of goals or a particular context (e.g. if one measure elicits a greater range of responses or shows clearer differentiation between the experiences of sub-populations of interest). There is also a risk in some contexts that people developing measures will promote their own tools disproportionately, with insufficient justification, for the reputational or financial gain that can be associated with the widespread adoption of measures, but we will not consider that further here.

We recognize the value of attempting to ensure that any definitions and linked metrics are somehow valid and reliable. Care should be taken not to use specious, overly simplistic or idiosyncratic definitions, and even if improvement researchers and practitioners shouldn't set their hopes on securing a single true definition and metric, there might be valuable work in identifying key features of quality concepts and distinguishing better from worse definitions and metrics – some of which may be context specific and others more generic. This will likely link into more pragmatic work to secure shared definitions for coordinated action across teams and organizations. We think, however, that there are serious limits to the value of trying to prove or disprove different definitions or attempting to work out the single best way of defining and measuring quality concepts, which are complex normative healthcare values. In practice, efforts to settle on a definition once and for all are liable to add yet another definition to the pile, rather than be universally accepted and consign all others to the archive.

We highlight two reasons for thinking that the search for the single best or true definition or metric for quality concepts is likely to be misguided. The first, which reflects a point made in Chapter 3 about quality as an overarching idea, is that different definitions and measures of any of the dimensions of quality are liable to highlight different aspects of a broad concept, often relative to particular purposes, rather than defining the 'whole' concept once and for all. This includes, more obviously, context-specific definitions but also generic definitions. Secondly, definitions of quality concepts are normative, in the sense that they reflect particular visions of what matters and why, and what should be relatively prioritized. Closing down discussion about what matters by choosing to work with a single definition risks failing to recognize the range of legitimate and defensible perspectives on what good healthcare (or some still complex aspect of it) looks like. We develop these points in the next two sub-sections.

5.3.1 Partial definitions and open-ended concepts

As we have been illustrating, more context-specific and especially more specifically operationalized definitions and metrics of quality or quality dimensions are liable to capture just a small part of broader concepts that reflect something about good healthcare. And the looser and the more open to interpretation a concept is in the first place, the more likely specification is to be partial and limited. When frustration is expressed about the lack of clear definitions for broad normative concepts, and the difficulty of operationalizing or measuring things that are subject to a lot of contestation and vagueness, it can seem like a more specific, narrow definition and a defined metric are needed to give form and content to the larger, hazier idea. But there is another possibility: that things are the other way round. That is, it is the broader sense of the meaning and value of quality concepts that lends shape and plausibility to specific definitions and operational models; without this background value-context it is difficult to make sense of narrower interpretations. Different definitions and models emphasize and draw out a range of different conceptual features that come to the fore or acquire particular significance in different settings but may underplay others that are nonetheless important for understanding the value and character of the concept for healthcare. These definitions overlap and inter-refer and -relate in ways that conjure up a vaguer, compound concept without a clear essence or set of necessary and sufficient conditions. Particular operational or local definitions sit in relation to this broader background concept and draw their meaning and value from it. Seeing things this way round helps to elucidate why it might not be helpful to settle on a single clear, operational definition, even though such definitions can be useful for coordinating action. The idea that a single best definition or metric can and should be chosen once and for all obscures these richer background concepts and threatens to hollow out much of their subtlety and depth – which are plausibly the things that make them key dimensions of healthcare and important social values.

One way of elucidating the open-ended nature of concepts is via the idea of a 'family resemblance concept'. Family resemblance concepts cannot be expressed in terms of a single, identifiable essence that characterizes all and only instances of the concept. The canonical example of a family resemblance concept, discussed at length by Ludwig Wittgenstein in his *Philosophical Investigations*, is the concept 'game'.[13] Wittgenstein argues that there is no single quality possessed by all games – some games are competitive and others are not; some are played for fun and others for money or political gain; some involve strategy and structure while others are open and spontaneous. Qualities that are possessed by all games – they are all forms of human activity, for example – are liable to be so broad that they do not distinctively pick out 'game' vis-à-vis other concepts. This should not lead to the conclusion that the true characteristics of 'game' should be definitively identified, and people should cease to refer to anything without such characteristics as a game. Instead, Wittgenstein suggests, 'game' should be understood to reflect an overlapping patchwork or network of characteristics, which are respectively shared by some but not all instances thereof. Identifying whether a particular activity is a game involves thinking about how it relates to other games and whether, and to what extent, it shares characteristics with them. This includes considering whether it is in fact seen as or identified as a game by other English speakers – that is, what the patterns of use of the concept 'game' are in practice. The overlapping patchwork that characterizes family resemblance concepts also implies that they do not have clearly defined or hard edges – some other activities and entities may share certain of the characteristics typical of games and not be games themselves. Distinguishing concepts and their appropriate use involves, then, not just conceptual analysis but also observation of competent language users and, moreover, being a competent language user oneself.

This suggests that, in many cases, the operational definitions and specifications of dimensions of quality that we have been discussing in this chapter should not be thought of as 'definitions' per se, at least insofar as this implies they are overarching and definitive characterizations. Instead, they could be thought of more like exemplars that, when taken together, identify and characterize the broader concept. This is perhaps easier to see in relation to specifications of quality dimensions that have been developed for and used in quite specific and contextualized purposes, but it can also apply more generally. For example, whether definitions of health equality emphasize access to healthcare, broader opportunities for health, measured health or wellbeing status, some other currency of distributive equality, or relational considerations, will likely depend on who and what the definition is for and what their scope of influence is (or is perceived to be). A model of equality that emphasizes equal access to healthcare may be useful to a healthcare service manager with decision-making power about resource allocation and service design who is trying to ensure that their services are available and accessible to all those who need them. A model that emphasizes equal health and well-being status may be more useful to policymakers trying to think at a population-wide health system level about how to relatively prioritize and allocate resources between different services, including balancing preventative, primary and secondary care; home-, community- and hospital-based care; and so on. These need not be thought to clash but rather to reflect the divergent demands and characteristics of different parts of healthcare systems and roles within them. Rather than seeing these different accounts as competing definitions, they can be seen as scope-limited examples of what equality might involve and demand in different settings and with different purposes in view.

This example begins to expose why, just as at the level of 'overall' quality, closing down the definitions of quality concepts may not be very helpful. Different definitions and metrics can reflect different purposes – whether institutional, sectoral or reflecting different visions of why health is important and what healthcare is for. These need not necessarily be seen as problematic conflicts – the different roles adopted by different healthcare professionals, including various clinical, strategic and operational roles – will enable and require them to think about and bring about good healthcare in quite different ways. Specific definitions often do not purport or aim to be universal and are often quite limited in their scope and ambitions. And where they do appear or even claim to be universal, this can implicitly reflect a more limited set of purposes and concerns, such as a particular institutional or professional framing.

5.3.2 Normative definitions and essentially contested concepts

The normativity of definitions makes claims that one definition is 'better' than others difficult to adjudicate and liable to contestation. We have highlighted and will now elaborate two ways in which operational definitions of dimensions of quality are normative: insofar as they (a) reflect different possible interpretations of a value concept and (b) can be used to pursue or promote different values.

First, then, definitions are normative because they reflect different interpretations of a normative concept. Whether equality (for example) is best understood in terms of access or outcomes, distributively or relationally, in relation to groups or individuals is not a matter of fact that can be discerned by research or observation. Such claims are value claims about what matters and why, which are justified by moral or conceptual argument (or underpinned by ethical and conceptual assumptions, if justification is not attempted). At best, descriptive claims can be made about what the majority of people think a quality concept such as equality comprises, or how people talk about it in practice, but further normative assumptions or claims are required to show that these findings tell us about the best or most appropriate way of using and defining these concepts. The normativity of definitions does not make it impossible to show that some are better than others, but the nature of this demonstration will in part depend on the validity and convincingness of arguments – that is, the extent to which people are in fact convinced by them – which itself is liable to be highly contestable.

The intractability of this normative disagreement suggests that it might be helpful to think of quality concepts as what W. B. Gallie calls 'essentially contested concepts'.[14] Gallie notes that some concepts are subject to seemingly irresolvable disagreement, with different uses being invoked by and serving different-but-related functions for different groups of people. This account resonates with, and extends and elucidates, what we referred to in Section 5.2 as the 'inherently interpretative' nature of at least some quality concepts. Gallie's examples include concepts like 'art' and 'democracy' but also plausibly could encompass central healthcare values such as 'efficiency', 'safety', 'respect' and 'care'. Gallie argues that disagreement and continued reflection on the meaning of some concepts are not just inevitable but also in some sense desirable. Disagreement about these concepts helps us to better understand their ethical and social significance and to develop and refine the values that they reflect. Debating the meaning of democracy or art is one way of grappling with the existential issues that we face individually and collectively and helps us to better understand how to conduct ourselves. Gallie argues that the proper use of these 'essentially contested concepts' inevitably involves endless disagreement about their proper uses.

Gallie suggests five constitutive characteristics of an essentially contested concept: (I) it is 'appraisive', meaning that it identifies the achievement of some valued thing; (II) the achievement is internally complex, attributed holistically or evaluatively rather than on the grounds of one consistent and easily identifiable factor; (III) explanations of its worth include reference to the respective contributions of its various parts, but there are different plausible descriptions of the importance and contributions of these different parts to its worth; (IV) the accredited achievement is open to modification in light of changing circumstances and such modification cannot be predicted in advance; (V) each party recognizes the fact that its own use of the concept is contested by other parties and each has some appreciation of the different criteria that the other parties claim to be applying. Quality concepts very plausibly possess these characteristics, being appraisive, evaluative, able to be described in different ways and responsive to circumstances. Disagreement and reflection on the meaning of these concepts, and the different ways of characterizing them, plausibly help us to think about what healthcare and health systems are for, and to consider the range of perspectives on this. A clear upshot of this would be that closing down disagreement and contextual variation in the definition and measurement of quality concepts would be inappropriate – though this is not to say that every proposed definition or characterization is valuable or should be promoted.

The second way in which definitions are normative is insofar as they serve normative purposes. Definitions and models are used to guide practice and improvement activities and so have the potential to shape healthcare systems and society more broadly, even if this isn't an explicit intention of their designers. The more immediate purposes served by a particular definition of person-centredness, for example, might include helping patients to better manage their condition at home, or finding treatment options that fit well with a patient's lifestyle and commitments, or trying to ensure that patients feel respected and listened to. These will reflect and embody a particular vision of what healthcare is *for*, suggesting, perhaps, a concern with broader well-being as well as the effective biomedical management of pathologies and clinical symptoms; a concern to minimize the burden of disease and healthcare on patients; a concern with efficient use of public funding and healthcare resources; and so on. Both the more proximate and the more remote purposes are normative insofar as they reflect different ideas of what the function and scope of healthcare ought to be; the values that healthcare ought to promote and embody; and notions of right and wrong intention and action. Crucially, there can be different valid and, to some extent, parallel visions of the function, scope and priorities of healthcare, not only because decision-making and creative power are distributed across the system, rather than centralized, but also because the health system and its component subsystems have and serve multiple co-existing functions.

5.4 Epistemic humility and sceptical calculative cultures

We have suggested that the field of healthcare improvement is strengthened when it embraces the open-endedness and variability entailed by the underlying normativity of quality concepts. Our argument is not that efforts towards 'pinning down' usable concepts through forms of operationalization and measurement should be abandoned and replaced by the unqualified assertion that quality is wholly interpretative and relative. Rather we welcome the commitment to conceptual clarity and rigour but argue that it can proceed in a hybrid fashion – both recognizing a role for operational definitions and, at the same time, combining that with explicit attention to the normativity of quality concepts and the multiple and multi-valent ways they can be deployed. This combination has the potential to help ensure that the pragmatic advantages of operational definitions and measures are retained while limiting the dangers arising from their being inevitably reductive, partial and selective, and thereby also potentially more favourable to some people, services and interests. A crucial component of the rigorous use of tools is to be clear about their limitations and more precisely to judge their utility and impacts against a rich nexus of evaluative and ethical concerns. We have suggested in the previous section that a first step in accepting that the open-ended, plural and contested nature of quality concepts can be unproblematic is to recognize that these characteristics occur routinely in the way language operates outside of technical contexts. A possible second step is to note that improvers do not have to be wedded to singular accounts of quality or even single toolkits of quality concepts as somehow unassailably 'correct' but can perfectly well 'mix and match' the concepts they use. Being critically reflective about the evaluative and ethical implications of the concepts and other tools that are in use, including the ways in which these are being, or might be, creatively combined, are key elements of what we are calling normatively conscious improvement work.

If improvers want to assess healthcare services in terms of complex, normative and socially significant values, they shouldn't expect there to be an easy or obvious way of measuring and making assessments about these values. Contestation, disagreement and high levels of contextual and interpretive variation should be expected. Indeed, we have suggested that sometimes disagreement can be a central feature of important social values and central to their being promoted and enacted well. In this concluding section, we offer if not a complete remedy then something of a salve. We encourage those involved in healthcare improvement activities to get comfortable with a degree of uncertainty and imprecision in operational definitions and measurement work, and to see measurement and measured change as tools for improvement rather than improvement ends in themselves. Uncertainty about the adequacy or limitations of a particular definition or measure shouldn't be thought to be a problem, but rather a sign that the systems and processes under consideration in any healthcare improvement efforts are extremely complex and can't be fully captured by a series of reductive metrics or analyses. We argue that would-be improvers should adopt an attitude of epistemic humility and a certain degree of caution with respect to the measurement of quality concepts, and we draw on Dane Pflueger's idea of a 'skeptical calculative culture' to suggest one possible approach.[15]

While the use of shared definitions and measures of quality concepts brings practical benefits of coordination, the reasons against either assuming that one well-established set is fully adequate or trying to identify a single best alternative when many are being proposed leave improvers with the prospect of having to live with uncertainty about the validity or adequacy of definitions and measures of healthcare quality and its dimensions. The arguments in this and the previous chapter suggest that, because of the high levels of interpretability and variability in quality concepts, improvement claims based on particular definitions and metrics will always reflect a particular interpretation and perspective on the healthcare systems, services and instances of care being assessed, and any suggestion that a definition or assessment is the 'best', or perhaps even 'good' or 'better', will be contestable. Moreover, we have argued that those involved in improvement projects cannot just rely on the definitions and measures of quality concepts that have been most used by others, but must reflect on how best to characterize, operationalize and measure the features of good healthcare in their particular context and given their purposes. If they don't do this, they will risk making improvement claims that are based on inappropriate conceptions of healthcare quality, do not reflect their purposes or mischaracterize the relevant features of the environment in question. The view we are recommending here might seem to produce an unfortunate state of affairs, not just because it introduces uncertainty to claims about quality and improvement, but also because it generates additional, and perhaps unwelcome, workload for would-be improvers. We think there is, however, reason to take a more optimistic attitude towards the uncertainties and open-endedness of improvement in the face of conceptual pluralism.

While the variety of ways of defining and measuring quality concepts does generate a degree of uncertainty about quality and improvement claims, this is not grounded in a lack of knowledge about these concepts but rather reflects their conceptual complexity and richness. The uncertainty and imprecision are to some extent inevitable and inherent to any attempt to operationalize these concepts. The social and ethical value of quality concepts is partly tied to their wide interpretability – that is, they capture something that is undeniably important, but important in different ways for different people, scenarios and systems. The uncertainty around their definition and measurement reflects genuine pluralism and irresolvable ambiguity in relation to knowledge claims about these concepts. And this is no bad thing. Precise and certain knowledge claims are useful if and when there are precise and certain things to know. In absence of these, they are liable to be precisely and certainly wrong.

How, then, should complex, normative concepts be approached, particularly when they are to be used in practical assessments and decision-making? We suggest that *epistemic humility* is a crucial idea for understanding and managing the uncertainties arising in these settings. Epistemic humility is a virtue that reflects a critical, questioning attitude towards one's 'cognitive repertoire', involving critical reflection on one's beliefs and belief systems, recognition of the limits of one's cognitive capacities and one's biases, acknowledgement of the defeasibility and uncertainty of particular beliefs, and willingness to change or moderate one's beliefs where appropriate.[16] Because the specification or measurement of complex, normative concepts is partial, perspectival and often involves a series of casual or associative claims relating to proxies or nearby concepts, claims about 'improvement' or performance in relation to such concepts should be made with epistemic humility, and caution should be exercised in making definitive claims on the basis of measures. Claims about the 'efficiency' or 'person-centredness' of services, for example, should be understood to be partial and provisional, insofar as they reflect a particular perspective on those services, incorporate certain sources and types of data, and are made at a particular point in time by individuals who bring their own interests, values and purposes to the activities of measurement and assessment.

At this point, practically minded readers might be thinking that this is all very well but those who are in the field designing, developing and trying to improve healthcare and healthcare systems want to make good decisions. That might seem like an impossible goal in light of so much uncertainty, epistemic humility notwithstanding. The idea is not, however, that some claims made about the quality of health services cannot be judged more valid, or informative, or in some way better than others. Rather, we are suggesting that even reflective and well-justified measurements and claims should not be taken as certain or conclusive assessments, but rather as information that contributes to more holistic claims about when and whether healthcare and healthcare systems are 'good' and 'better'.

One way of managing the limited and uncertain nature of definitions, measurements and claims relating to quality concepts is to develop what Dane Pflueger calls a 'skeptical calculative culture'.[17] Pflueger recognizes the importance of measurement and accounting in healthcare quality and healthcare improvement but also understands the limitations of particular measures and measurement approaches, and the dangers of relying on reductive accounts of healthcare systems for making claims about quality and deciding to change processes and activities. He introduces the idea of a 'skeptical calculative culture' to characterize institutional approaches and attitudes that treat particular measurements or pieces of evidence not as the underlying reality about quality, but as possible indications of quality. Measurements of healthcare services, within such systems, are treated not as answers to questions about quality, but as inputs into deliberations and discussions about quality and its dimensions. Such cultures are sceptical insofar as individual measures are treated as defeasible and partial, as contributing to but not exhausting more holistic judgements and evaluative assessments about quality. And they are calculative insofar as they value measurement as a crucial decision-making tool and are concerned to generate valid measurements and make judicious use of metrics and evidence-gathering tools. It's worth noting, however, that it is not only quantitative data that are treated as indicators of quality and used as the basis for deliberative discussions and more holistic evaluations – qualitative evidence, absence of evidence, known unknowns and tacit knowledge may also play a role alongside quantitative evidence and analysis in quality assessments. Using a variety of different indicators and measures in parallel, accepting that each is partial, imperfect and defeasible, will allow for the generation of a more nuanced and inclusive – though not exhaustive – picture of these aspects of healthcare quality. Because these accounts are likely to include internal inconsistencies and uncertainties, they cannot be used directly to resolve questions of what is better or what to do. They can, however, help to guide and inform our judgements in a way that is evidence-based but not simplistic.

This vision of a sceptical calculative culture expresses an important idea that we want to reiterate: measurement and different forms of evidence that might be gathered about healthcare quality and its dimensions are not in themselves the reality of healthcare quality, nor can assessments of quality be read off them directly. Rather, they are tools that contribute to and help people to make more holistic and evaluative assessments of quality. Failure to recognize this amounts to a failure to see healthcare quality and quality dimensions as the *normative* concepts that they are – as telling us something about what good healthcare looks like and how healthcare and healthcare services ought to be. Seeing measurement as an end in itself, rather than means to an end, in relation to healthcare quality and healthcare improvement, frames improvement as a *technical* exercise. It reflects an assumption that improvement involves understanding the extent to which healthcare services have certain defined characteristics and taking steps to ensure that they do, or do not, continue to have them. The kind of sceptical calculative culture that we are endorsing instead emphasizes the broader aim of *good* healthcare, and so demands continual (or at least periodic) reflection on whether and why particular measured characteristics are helpful indicators of values such as quality dimensions.

For the avoidance of doubt, we stress that the points we are making apply to quality dimensions that are typically thought of as 'harder' as well as those typically thought of as 'softer'. For, as we illustrated in Chapter 4, the process of operationalizing 'harder' quality dimensions is underpinned by interpretative and normative judgements, and these dimensions are also subject to wide variability, such that those seeking to make quality and improvement assessments in these areas also need to manage uncertainty and conflicting evidence and measurements. A humble and cautious approach to measurement and making quality claims has the potential to be more burdensome on healthcare staff and services than the alternative approach of treating simple measures as sufficient for making quality assessments, but the more reflective approach that we are advocating for will better accommodate the range of values and perspectives inherent to healthcare and to improvement activities. There is little point in improvement activities if they are simplistic and reductive, and do not reflect a rich account of healthcare processes and their multiple underlying functions and purposes.

What we are advocating here involves deliberate, reflective, self-conscious engagement with normative complexity. This leaves plenty of space for scientific-technical ways of thinking about healthcare improvement but simply makes these constantly subject to critical scrutiny including ethical checks and balances. Deciding whether healthcare is of good quality or is being improved always rests on value judgements including the ethical work of somehow holding together a range of concerns, perspectives and interests rather than simply thinking about the maximization of outcomes in some sharply defined way.

PART THREE

MAKING ETHICS VISIBLE

6 ETHICS AND HEALTHCARE IMPROVEMENT

We now turn to a sustained consideration of a theme that we have touched upon in the preceding chapters – the ethics of healthcare improvement. For brevity we call this focus 'improvement ethics'. While Part 2 focused mainly on conceptual issues and highlighted the ways in which claims about what is good or better in healthcare are value laden, Part 3 focuses on practical ethical issues faced by those involved in improvement activities. The two chapters in this part of the book cover similar ground but have different emphases. Chapter 6 sets out and illustrates the range of values at play in improvement approaches and the complexity of improvement ethics. Chapter 7 asks how improvers manage, and could better manage, the ethical challenges of the field and considers some of the practical and analytical resources available to address ethical issues.

Recognizing the normative complexity of healthcare improvement, we have argued, makes thinking about ethics central to undertaking improvement. In practice, much of that thinking is currently implicit and uncharted and we suggest that there needs to be more emphasis on deliberate, explicit and self-conscious discussion of ethics. The suggestion is not just that addressing ethics is an important but relatively neglected sub-theme but that it is core to strengthening improvement thinking more generally. Attending to ethics helps to bring into focus what improvers are doing, and the balancing acts this entails, and supports a shift towards richer, more open-ended, and plural conceptions of and approaches to evaluation.

In previous chapters we have shown how the concerns of the improvement field and the concerns of ethics are closely intertwined.

Healthcare improvement is meant to increase the likelihood of valuable healthcare processes and goods being enacted and achieved. Even when improvers discuss their objectives in technical terms, it is reasonable to imagine they are fuelled by motivations that can also be described in ethical terms. More specific resonances between improvement and ethics can be seen in relation to quality dimensions. The goal of increasing efficiency and the patient safety agenda of trying to reduce the overall harms caused by healthcare are often subject to broadly consequentialist models of evaluation – at least when these aims are operationalized in more reductive ways to support quantitative estimation of quality gains. By contrast the values of person-centredness and equality – and in particular efforts to ensure that people are 'seen', respected and treated appropriately and fairly as individuals and groups – complicate and suggest limits to maximizing tendencies in consequentialist thinking. We have also argued that different quality dimensions cannot be neatly separated out but overlap and need to be thought about in combination. What we have illustrated in the chapters in Part 2 is that as improvers draw on and specify various constructions of quality to direct or assess their efforts, they are, in effect, articulating valued ends and weighing different value considerations together and thereby implicitly asking and answering ethical questions.

Much of our discussion has stressed that constructions of 'improvements' (the 'what') are laden with values and ethical assumptions, but it is equally important to highlight that improvement approaches and activities (the 'how') also require ethical attention. Like any kind of activity, improvement policies and practices can produce unforeseen harms and commit wrongs such as disrespecting and undermining people and being unfair. The fact that such practices are aimed at improvement and may be 'doing good' does not change this, except perhaps it should make us extra cautious about what might happen (no doubt unintentionally) under the umbrella of benign motivation. But there is much more to the ethics of improvement than determining what maximizes service 'outputs' and minimizes harmful 'side effects'. For example, there are procedural questions about what forms and levels of agreement, and from whom, ought to prefigure and accompany service change. These are analogous to those raised in longstanding debates in clinical care about the need for people to consent to clinical interventions. And there are questions about who should be consulted and how to determine how to characterize good and bad practice and outcomes in order to evaluate the success of interventions.

In this chapter we consider what becomes visible when would-be improvers shift the emphasis from implicit to explicit thinking about ethics – thus sketching out an imagined field of 'improvement ethics'. We start by briefly illustrating the kinds of issues that might arise for improvement ethics from within healthcare practice and, specifically, from the point of view of one imagined practitioner. This illustrative case will serve to show how wide-ranging and diffuse ethical issues can be in the improvement field, how ethical issues can be 'nested' within one another and how questions about specific practices are likely to involve consideration of more far-reaching questions and contexts. We then 'zoom out' from healthcare practice and compare 'improvement ethics' with other areas in healthcare ethics. We argue that improvement ethics has overlaps with clinical ethics and research ethics but especially – we will stress – public health ethics. We suggest that the relative scale and 'landscape shaping' aspects of improvement work, emphasized by the comparison with public health, raise distinctive ethical challenges. We discuss two sets of challenges: first, those relating to how to prioritize different improvement activities relative to one another and, second, those relating to the coordination of activities and responsibilities across differently placed actors in a complexly interwoven field.

The initial impression created by unpacking these nested layers of possible contention and debate is that bringing ethical issues into the light simply makes reasoning about improvement unmanageable. As we will set out more fully in Chapter 7, however, we envisage a process that is positive, productive and consistent with the practical demands of healthcare. Responsible healthcare improvement does not avoid explanatory complexity or practical empirical complications but aims to acknowledge and address them in order to strengthen and extend the practice of improvement. The same can and should apply to normative complexity and practical ethical challenges.

6.1 Illustrating improvement ethics

We start from the position of one imagined healthcare actor, Fatima. Fatima is a paediatric hospital consultant who has developed an interest in improving healthcare. What aspects of her work might be relevant to improvement ethics? We briefly review four possible examples.

Some of Fatima's improvement-related work is relatively continuous with her normal or routine professional practice:

1   *Clinical handovers*: Fatima is collaborating with nursing colleagues on a local initiative which involves trialling a revised protocol to improve clinical handovers.[1]

2   *National care standards*: She is participating in, and complying with procedures in, a national programme designed to monitor and enhance care standards based upon officially authorized clinical standards and performance indicators.[2]

Other aspects of her 'improvement-related' work are less continuous with normal professional practice:

3   *Poverty screening*: Fatima is part of a group developing and applying a system of screening for markers of social deprivation for families, allied to new forms of referral to social and welfare services.[3]

4   *Paediatric professionalism*: She is engaged in a broader project – working with networks of colleagues in a range of institutions regionally and nationally – to rethink paediatric professionalism with the aim that it becomes better 'joined up' with broader social services and agendas and more effectively responsive to the social determinants of health and well-being.[4]

Even these few examples are enough to indicate some of the kinds of ethical questions that can arise in relation to improvement-related activities.

Although she is unlikely to think in terms of ethical theory, many kinds of ethical concerns (and vocabularies) will likely be relevant to Fatima.[5] These include the quantities and qualities of different kinds of good and bad things brought about by given actions (as highlighted by consequentialism); any norms or rules that determine what people ought to do or not to do (deontology); and desirable character qualities that underpin the capacity of individuals to both see and practise what counts as wise and good conduct (virtue theory). They may also include the central importance of: connections between, and the mutual constitution of, people (communitarianism and feminist ethics); choice and individual autonomy (liberalism); and equality (egalitarianism). Fatima's potential concerns might be crudely summarized as about goals, obligations, dispositions and relationships: (a) what range of benefits (and harms) is the unit trying to bring about (or avoid); (b) what duties do members of the team owe to patients and each other, either because of role-specific requirements or just as people; (c) what are desirable character qualities for colleagues to have or develop; and (d) might these various concerns, at least sometimes, be best understood and approached through the lens of protecting and cultivating good relationships between people? This range of relevant concerns underlines the extent to which 'outputs' and 'consent', two key considerations for health services, are too limited a framing for a fully rounded improvement ethics. Fatima may also be keen to ask whether people are being treated fairly, whether diverse identities are being recognized and respected and whether, and how far, everyone is meaningfully participating in shaping the environment.

The questions raised by these concerns are not very different from the questions many improvers feel bound to ask of themselves in any case, although, of course, they may not associate them with the language of ethics. For each example there are the ethical questions we summarized in the introduction as about the 'what' and the 'how' – questions about purposes including visions of healthcare, and questions about processes and relationships. The former set of issues relates to ends. They call for judgements about whether what results from improvement activities is good rather than bad, or more likely (and more challenging) whether good consequences 'outweigh' bad ones, both in theory and in practice. The latter set of issues concerns improvement methods and ask improvers to determine whether the way a desired improvement is pursued is otherwise ethically acceptable or desirable, or how they can best navigate the ethical compromises involved. This two-fold way of presenting things seems relatively clear and tidy, but practical examples open up a very wide range of relevant considerations.

In the case of Fatima's *clinical handovers* project, for example, thinking about the 'what' would include asking about the possible purposes and uses of handovers and their unintended as well as intended effects. For example, handovers should draw attention to salient issues in particular patients' care, thereby making it more likely that these will be appropriately attended to by incoming clinical staff and helping to ensure that care and communication are consistent. But, in practice, there is a risk that handovers can give a false sense of security to incoming clinical staff, with the issues mentioned by their colleagues being treated as if they were a relatively complete checklist, leading to emerging or previously unidentified issues being indirectly downplayed. Improvers looking to change things thus need to be mindful not only of their intended goals but of the potential unintended costs of change. They need to ask what valuable things might be unintentionally lost in moving away from the previous practice model and to consider how (through what lenses and methods) the change is being mapped, monitored and measured – do these neglect aspects of quality or fail to do justice to the concerns they are meant to capture?

With regard to the 'how' of the *clinical handovers* project, Fatima and her colleagues might ask who is involved in designing, enacting and evaluating the change, and take seriously how staff (and families) who are affected by the envisaged change are being treated. For example, how does it impact on staff workload, or the way workload is counted? How does it affect staff scope for exercising autonomy, initiative and creativity in conducting handovers? More broadly, how far are staff being pressurized and/or meaningfully consulted with to achieve the change? This latter concern, which we can label in general terms as about 'forms of influence' over people, is of widespread relevance and importance, alongside the concern with evaluating and weighing the results of change. The 'what' and 'how' emphases may be difficult to disentangle. A concern with forms of influence may reflect an interest in respecting staff, ensuring their well-being, and maintaining their professional discretion and autonomy – valuing these in their own right. But a failure to attend to these factors and to consider them in the design of improvement projects might also lead to unintended effects. Disgruntled, disengaged or overworked staff may be unable or unwilling to participate fully in improvement projects and, in extremis, may even try to undermine or sabotage them. An interest in successful outcomes of improvement projects will therefore also justify an interest in the acceptability of the process.

One of the advantages of conceiving of the evaluation of improvement in terms of ethics is that it stimulates more holistic and pluralistic approaches to evaluation than the relatively narrow and specified frameworks often required by managerial systems and some influential models of research. Such frameworks can provide a useful discipline but do not always support the open-ended interrogation of practice that many healthcare professionals welcome. There is not always a sharp contrast to be made here though. For example, some technically framed studies of clinical handover improvement are relatively broad ranging – looking at providing more time with patients, the improvement of communication with patients and families, as well as reduction in medical errors and other patient safety issues and metrics.[6] Nonetheless Fatima may well be inclined to set these issues in an even wider context. If she is ethically conscientious and operates with a relatively open-ended concern with getting the unit to 'work well' – to do the 'right things' and have the 'right culture' – she will want any improvement to contribute to rather than impair that aspiration.

As we have been stressing, ethical issues are routinely obscured by technical discourses that narrow the gaze. This effect can be compounded by the way improvement objectives and activities might, in practice, be defined by the institutional agendas and wider service priorities, rather than the needs of specific patient groups or locally informed judgements. The *national care standards* example is a case in point. Fatima and her colleagues are regularly collecting and reporting data about compliance with specific care standards and protocols as part of a national programme. This might reasonably be assumed to be a desirable and unproblematic activity. But it is not difficult to conceive of ways in which, on examination, it raises ethical concerns. Even supposing that the standards are each rigorously derived and appropriate there might be questions about whether other important things will be relatively sidelined or deprioritized by an emphasis on the standards. Or whether this standard-set is as good a fit for the distinctive population and communities served by Fatima's unit as it is for the majority of units. In addition, questions could be asked about the 'forms of influence' that are deployed in the programme. Are there institutional or professional incentives to comply with this form of monitoring and could that somehow distort the local 'attention economy' and the motivation of colleagues? What are the likely global unintended 'side effects' of some valued things, but not other valued things, being subject to institutional incentives?

In some cases it is possible that an impartial appraisal of an institutionally fostered improvement activity would conclude that, overall, it is harmful or even ethically wrong – if, for example, it has unintended or unanticipated effects that makes people's experiences worse, or if it is effectively unfair or disrespectful to some subset of people. This is not a purely hypothetical concern. The potential for limited institutional constructions of improvement to fall short, or even get in the way, of actual improvements has already been noted in the specific context of paediatric care,[7] and there are clear voices within the healthcare improvement community who articulate ways in which improvement activities can produce 'bad effects'.[8] A discussion amongst a group of reflective improvement professionals will elicit and exemplify a range of ways in which improvement efforts can go wrong and thereby raise ethical concerns: because, for example, they have the 'wrong aims' (ones judged too limited or taking services in the wrong direction); they adopt inappropriate approaches or models of practice, or mis-apply approaches; they waste resources (i.e. they have unjustified opportunity costs); they are burdensome to over-stretched (possibly already burnt-out) staff. These problems can easily be caused or exacerbated by institutional working conditions such as managerial pressures, time constraints, and inexperienced or unsupported staff.[9] We noted this internal scepticism in Chapter 1 and underline it here. It might be too obvious to be worth stating but perhaps it is too important not to state that just because something is conscientiously intended as an improvement it does not follow that it is a good thing.

The third and fourth examples of Fatima's improvement-related work mentioned above reflect a more revisionary perspective, one which attempts to look beyond prevailing institutional expectations. But, of course, they still raise ethical issues, which we briefly indicate here. Looking at the *poverty screening* example first: assuming the poverty screening 'works' in some sense – the challenges of deciding what this means were discussed in Chapter 2 – is it acceptable to raise socially invasive topics when families attend a secondary care clinic for what they might see as a purely disease-centred agenda or is it, on the contrary, irresponsible to regard people's experience of poverty as 'off-limits'?[10] The *paediatric professionalism* example raises a number of linked issues relating to the ethics of profession-building including the advantages and disadvantages of re-drawing boundaries between services and roles. For example, in what circumstances is the formal extension of professional roles and remits demanded? How far is it ethically problematic to encourage professional colleagues to take on responsibilities that they see as sitting outside their areas of specialist expertise? These are demanding questions. For example, they link to discussions in Chapter 5 about different possible conceptions of both person-centredness and equity and the ways that these dimensions of quality can be interpreted either in ways that can be accommodated within a delivery perspective or in ways that suggest revisionary actions are needed. These value-laden conceptual possibilities may lead to difficult deliberations and judgements about whether and why professional roles need to be reconceived, or whether key ambitions can instead be reflected in existing conventions and professional training with relatively minimal change.

Fatima's improvement-related work begins to illustrate the ethical challenges of improvement. The questions raised might be relatively commonplace. Comparable questions about balancing and trading off values form the basis of established discussions about case-based and principle-based decision-making in bioethics and public health ethics, for example. However, they are not amenable to easy answers. There may be some instances in which ethical issues are both manifest and relatively straightforward – for example, if a colleague lies purely for personal gain or is motivated to harm others. But most of the time things are far less clear-cut as there are relevant considerations that pull in different directions.

Thinking about the challenges facing one professional highlights the gap between relatively detached approaches to ethics (as found in much academic ethics) and ethics seen from the real-world standpoints of particular people. The former often do not focus on the position of specific actors but rather ask what ought to happen or be done in very general, and often abstract and impersonal, terms. This is only partially helpful for individuals who face the practical question of 'What falls to me – what ought I to do here and now?' Of course, actual healthcare professionals will not share Fatima's imagined improvement projects and professional identity but will nonetheless be able to map the approaches to ethical reasoning relevant to Fatima's examples onto their own. The examples we have given show that improvement ethics needs to encompass quite contrasting cases in terms of focus and scale – ranging from small projects in immediate clinical settings to expansive policy or context-shaping activities. Indeed, they illustrate that the former cannot be adequately tackled without some reference to the latter. To ask about improving a particular setting or range of practices is to raise questions about the broader social contexts and the background assumptions that shape settings and practices. Seriously addressing questions of improvement practice leads on to engagement with philosophical puzzles about healthcare. We develop this idea in the following sections as we continue our sketch of improvement ethics.

6.2 The relative distinctiveness of improvement ethics

We are not suggesting that ethics for improvement or improvers is, or should be, treated as a new specialist sub-field of applied ethics. We accept the argument others have made about the need to avoid a proliferation of such sub-fields, especially where there is no good reason to imagine that new theoretical lenses or methodologies are either required or available to underpin them.[11] In this section we suggest that, although it overlaps with both clinical ethics and research ethics, improvement ethics is more closely analogous to (and might plausibly even be seen as a branch of) public health ethics. This, we argue, is because engaging in improvement implies an element of scale which has rule-making and context-shaping effects. Improvement activities – and not only when they take a more 'revisionary' form – shape the landscapes in which others work and experience care, including by questioning the norms built into and cemented through existing practices.

6.2.1 Improvement in relation to clinical practice and research

The examples of Fatima's improvement work discussed in the previous section vary in scale but they all 'reach beyond' her own practice and endeavour to shape the conditions for a range of actors. They are continuous with but, in some respects, transcend the scope of clinical ethics. Within clinical professional ethics it is, at least sometimes, sufficient for clinicians to carefully think about a particular case and set of circumstances and come to the conclusion that it is justified to organize or enact care in a given way. But an aim to improve things calls for a different lens: it puts in place or supports arrangements with the intention that other people (possibly very many) are more likely to be organizing or enacting care in a given way. If this is a sensible characterization then it has substantial ethical relevance because it highlights that healthcare improvement is analogous to a policymaking or even legislative role, particularly in the requirement to think about scale and monitoring over time.

There is no sharp distinction between a health professional such as Fatima 'doing their job' and them engaging in improvement activities. This is because the ideas of professional practice and professionalism contain learning and capability building as an inherent part, and these are central to improvement discourses and ambitions. Learning is pursued and promoted by an individual's own education, training and professional development activities, but it often extends much wider than that and includes addressing the potential impact of working context: developing the institutional conditions and knowledge bases that enable individuals to do their work well and support the building of a 'learning culture'. In this general sense, improvement activities are intrinsic to professional practice. In broad terms what diverse improvement practices have in common is that they are rooted in a reflexive, evaluative and constructive orientation to healthcare. They involve the analysis of, or the undertaking of, systematic changes to the ways in which healthcare activities are organized and/or enacted. To the extent that clinical practitioners adopt this orientation to their work they are 'improvers' as well as clinicians.

This connects to an oft-cited idea in healthcare improvement circles that everyone in healthcare has two jobs: to do their work and to improve their work.[12] Healthcare workers will sometimes just be focused on tasks that need to be done and, necessarily, lean heavily on already established 'scripts'. But professionals such as Fatima could be seen as having two modes that exist alongside one another, with the more critical and reflective 'improvement' mode sometimes disappearing into the background and sometimes coming to the fore. If, as we have suggested, the field of healthcare improvement is concerned with systematic shared change, then not everything Fatima does to improve the way she does her job would fall into the field. Attending a course on communication skills and practising them so as to do a better job would not, in itself, count as a contribution to healthcare improvement. But where these kinds of changes are being deliberately recommended or otherwise supported within a service (and especially where they are being carefully monitored or even measured) they count as improvement activity and become a focus for improvement ethics.

This picture of improvement, which stresses reflexivity, evaluation and change at scale (to some degree), also highlights continuities and resemblances between improvement and research, most obviously research allied to service development. This comparison captures something valid about the field of healthcare improvement. First, people who are 'improvement researchers' make up a significant part of the field; second, it is typically taken for granted that improvement practice should be research-informed – that is, based on research studies or, at minimum, systematically collected data. This indicates a significant area of overlap between research ethics and improvement ethics.

However, there are strict limits to how far there is an equivalence here. Research is treated differently from most areas of healthcare practice. It is notable that extensive systems of research governance have been established and that it is an area where discussion of ethics is already established as a norm. Anyone wishing to undertake healthcare research takes it for granted that they need not only to think through the ethical issues their projects may entail but they must also subject themselves to official institutionalized forms of accountability to explain and defend their research choices, in the form of review by research ethics committees and monitoring of conformity to research ethics standards. Rightly or wrongly – and there are arguments for thinking this is sometimes overdone – research is treated as exceptional.[13] Probably the core reason for this exceptionalism is that any particular research study is regarded as effectively 'optional' in the sense that services exist (and continue) in parallel to it, so the research activities involve extra burdens, in terms of time, costs and risks, for patients and staff. These additional burdens can only be justified if there are good grounds for thinking that lines of research are worth doing and that studies are well designed to contribute to the relevant knowledge base. Institutional systems of research governance have been put in place to safeguard research standards and to protect the interests of patients and other stakeholders, including by limiting the extent to which the same people are subject to proliferating numbers of studies. There is certainly a case for treating some subset of improvement projects in broadly the same way as research projects, and we will discuss the institutional governance of research and its relevance to accountability for improvement projects further in Chapter 7.

But, more broadly, improvement is different from research. Research is primarily oriented towards knowledge production and improvement towards change, including knowledge utilization. One important distinction links into the discussion of day-to-day professionalism above: many aspects of improvement are non-optional but are necessarily embedded within practice and policymaking.[14] When any healthcare activity is planned, at micro-, meso- or macro-levels, thought must be given to whether the way in which it is organized and enacted will help make it good quality. These decisions are made constantly and often need to be revisited and remade on a regular, sometimes daily, basis as circumstances change. There is no meaningful sense in which this process is optional. In addition, although planning and organizing decisions should, where possible, be research-informed it does not make sense to expect every aspect of every relevant decision to be either a product of research or subject to research (at least in the conventional health services sense of empirical studies planned for knowledge generation). This is not solely for pragmatic reasons but also for ethical and conceptual reasons. The scale of research activity called for would be massively large to manage, the burdens of research on subjects would be unbearable and, in addition, there would be an indefinitely large number of ways of framing, posing, dividing up or aggregating relevant questions and approaches.

In order that healthcare services are no worse than, and ideally better than, the ones that were in place last year or last week, healthcare practitioners and improvers cannot decide on courses of action in wholly arbitrary ways. But research projects are not the only things that can be contrasted with arbitrariness. Healthcare decision-makers routinely take into account the experienced perceptions and reflections of practitioners, patients and others along with routine organizational data (the collection of which is loosely analogous to research), and much of this happens in informal organic ways rather than by the circumscribed approaches typical of health services research. In some respects, decisions may be less robust as a result – but not necessarily in all respects. More informal information gathering can sometimes access important insights that are difficult for research to reach. This might include things which, for various reasons, people think and talk about, but don't want to 'go on the record' with or formalize, as well as tacit knowledge about how institutions operate that is difficult to codify. Such factors might be crucial in determining, for example, the areas of focus for or broad direction of improvement activities. There could be a vague and near metaphorical sense of research where there is a closer equation between the requirements of improvement and research. Here 'research' might signify something like disciplined attention, thoughtful reflection and some degree of explicit, 'peer reviewable' or 'publicly auditable' thinking, but this vague sense is not what is conventionally understood, or regulated, as research.

6.2.2 Improvement in relation to public health

These parallels suggest that improvement ethics might be seen as closely allied to public health ethics (or perhaps even a branch of it). We start by briefly summarizing four parallels between improvement and public health and outlining their implications for ethics. First, public health – like healthcare improvement – is held together by a broad aim (improving the health of the public) rather than a clear-cut group of 'workers' or defined set of practices, although there are of course public health professionals, just as there are improvement professionals. Public health does include its 'own' characteristic practices such as vaccination, screening, health surveillance and public education, and research methods, in particular epidemiological approaches, but it also encompasses an indefinitely large set of activities and approaches. These arguably include those designed to underpin the suitability and good functioning of health services as one platform for protecting and promoting population health. This mirrors the loose grouping of improvers and improvement activities that healthcare improvement incorporates.

Second, in many instances public health interventions are not direct clinical interventions into people's bodies (although some are). Rather they are often targeted at changing the conditions of social life and action. That is, they may work through a range of 'forms of influence' – for example, legal requirements or constraints, financial dis/incentives, peer pressure, or other forms of encouragement or discouragement, including appeals to solidarity and provision of information or education. Similarly, improvement interventions often focus on changing attitudes and organizational processes rather than trying to implement or change clinical interventions directly.

Third, public health analysis and action can be more narrowly or broadly targeted – it can be focused on reducing the impact of a specific kind of disease or health risk (e.g. by interrupting transmission or by implementing more effective prevention and management policies) or it can be aimed at 'system strengthening' in a way that might have widespread benefits across a variety of conditions (e.g. by enhancing communication and intelligence sharing between different service strands). This distinction is sometimes described using the contrast of 'vertical' and 'horizontal' approaches – the former 'narrowing in' on specific areas of mortality and morbidity (such as obesity) and targeting the relevant sets of causes and policy responses; the latter aimed at reinforcing and developing social, policy and service infrastructures that underpin provision and care, and which have benefits across the board.[15] A similar (and similarly helpful) distinction has been applied to the healthcare improvement field between those aspects of practice that involve targeted 'interventions' and those that are directed more broadly at 'context-strengthening'.[16] (Fatima's local trial of a new *clinical handover* protocol could exemplify the former, and her broader *paediatric professionalism* project the latter, although like other individual projects or programmes, both can involve a combination of targeted and context-strengthening elements.)

Fourth, public health involves not only diffused agency but also, it follows, diffused responsibility. Large numbers of people, located in very many contrasting settings and roles, play a part in public health, both as sources of potential interventions and in terms of having their agency implicated. The implementation of no-smoking policies in restaurants will serve as an example. Governments and local policymakers, public educators and mass media have a role, but so too do restaurant owners, staff and individual diners who have a de facto say in how to interpret, apply and follow such a policy and whether this happens with or without degrees of resistance. These levels of diffused agency produce significant puzzles about how to ascribe responsibility when things go either smoothly or badly. This has been labelled the 'problem of many hands' and recognized as significant within the field of healthcare improvement.[17] How can improvement action be coordinated and who is responsible for doing what, including initiating and coordinating action, when improvement involves contributions and engagement from so many? There is an obvious danger that if everyone is held responsible for some desired change, no-one takes responsibility in practice – a familiar feature of everyday social coordination.

The correspondences between public health and healthcare improvement arise in part from their epistemic similarities and the analogous hurdles they face. More specifically, they both work 'at scale' and thus have to deal with relatively open-ended systems and explanatory complexity. In other words, both public health and improvement involve developing practical interventions but in complex systems in which it is difficult to isolate and track lines of cause and effect and to generalize about 'what works' and what is valuable from one setting to another. These parallels shed light on the challenges facing improvement ethics. They help explain why it is a 'big subject' and, in particular, the high level of indeterminacy in the area. Unless improvement is characterized from an extremely narrow interpretation of a delivery standpoint – such that the sole job of improvement is to help services 'work' in the technical sense of reliably replicating whatever they are meant to do – then improvers must confront quite general questions about the nature and function of healthcare. To start with, there are ethical puzzles about what an improver's purposes and priorities should be because there are various visions of good healthcare within which a range of competing goods are differently constructed and weighted. The choice of possible approaches is equally open-ended, including very different kinds of activities on multiple axes and levels both vertically and horizontally. Improvement practice can deploy a range of 'forms of influence' – more or less 'top-down', 'bottom-up', coercive, enabling, collaborative and so on – and the ethics of legal compulsion, managerial targets, peer support, co-production and other such mechanisms each require separate consideration. The public health parallels open up very general ethical puzzles about both 'what' and 'how' that we discuss further in the next two sections. They also highlight the ways in which normative complexity reflects, and interacts with, explanatory complexity, which we return to in the final section.

There are many topics in improvement ethics that we could discuss in more detail, but we have chosen here to introduce two sets of questions – about priorities (in Section 6.3) and 'who does what?' (in Section 6.4) – to illustrate the kinds of tensions and normative complexities that we have been discussing. These questions have central relevance to a broad range of improvement activities and projects and illustrate the importance of navigating improvement ethics in practice.

6.3 Priorities, thresholds and timescales

We have used the comparison with public health to sketch out some of the distinctive character and shape of improvement ethics. One prominent theme is the scope for debate about healthcare purposes and hence the 'what' of improvement. This obviously connects with the question of 'priority setting' – a well-known aspect of public health and healthcare ethics. Of all the improvements that might be made and to which improvers could devote research and time, effort and resource, which ones should come first?

More precisely – given that improvers can and no doubt should aim to achieve many things simultaneously – which 'bundles of improvements' should (differently placed) actors prioritize? As is often the case, a broad framework might be assembled but that is not the same as providing a real-world answer, which would require the practical, contextual interpretation and application of any such framework. A broad framework might involve asking, at least:

- what kinds of improvements might make the most substantial difference to people's health outcomes, care relationships and experiences;

- how good or bad care standards currently are in the domains addressed by potential improvements;

- how well-evidenced, feasible and acceptable the relevant approaches and methods are;

- how much of which kinds of resources including the necessary expertise are available; and

- which groups of people might receive benefits or risk being relatively neglected.

Each strand of this simple framework raises complex theoretical and empirical questions that are also normatively complex and can lead to considerable contestation. And, moreover, combining the kinds of guidance that could be gleaned from each strand (assuming useful answers could be constructed in each case) would also generate ethical dilemmas. For example, how far can worse health outcomes be compensated for by improvements in health equity? And to what extent should improvement activities in areas of very poor performance be prioritized when larger health gains could be made by focusing on areas with average performance?

Here we focus on two linked issues to illustrate the deep-seated contestability of priority setting: different healthcare quality thresholds and different timescales. These are also significant in public health and are arguably core to the improvement field. We start with the question of thresholds. Put crudely, how much is the goal of improvement to make bad care adequate, to make adequate care better or to make good care excellent, and how should improvers divide time and other resource between these? There are, of course, a range of possible threshold levels here, and these are sometimes crystallized into simple descriptors by inspection or ranking exercises. For example, the Care Quality Commission, England's independent health regulator, uses four summary descriptors for the services they inspect: 'outstanding, good, requires improvement and inadequate'.[18]

These kinds of threshold levels have prima facie ethical relevance, reflecting widely held prioritarian or sufficientarian concerns with focusing on areas where things are particularly bad first. Assuming all else is equal, it is plausible to suppose that there is less of a moral imperative to try and shift a service from 'good' to 'outstanding' than an equivalent service from 'inadequate' to 'adequate'. There might also – to show the linkage with timescales – be reason to think that there is less 'urgency' in the former case. After all a good service should surely be relatively welcomed and celebrated. There may be scope to improve it further, but it is not obvious that this needs to be done today – and especially not if the time and resources could be used to improve things in areas where standards are worse and where, we should not forget, real people may be suffering unnecessarily. This is not, incidentally, intended as a wholesale rejection of an idea like 'continuous quality improvement' but it does suggest that this idea needs some critical scrutiny. Supposing that a healthcare team has taken a service from inadequate to just adequate, there can be every reason to press on with improvements and no good reason to slow down, especially if there is momentum and enthusiasm within the team and the improvement activities have incurred one-off setup costs. This does not, however, rule out the possibility that at some point it might be justifiable for the quest for further improvements to be slowed, whilst (and perhaps to enable) being mindful about maintaining high standards.

The apparent ethical significance of thresholds for prioritization may be one reason for the relative prominence that is often attached to 'safety' in improvement discourses and practices. Whilst it is possible to mount a sociological critique of the relative prominence of safety in improvement agendas – for example, as reflecting a particularly well-established and vocal 'patient safety industry' – this would not seem to get to the essence of things. Rather healthcare professionals and policymakers have a longstanding, deeply embedded commitment to providing services which do not cause harm to people. A harmful service is uncontroversially a bad service. Obviously some harms are unavoidable effects of treatments and interventions but, as discussed in Chapter 4, patient safety focuses on avoidable iatrogenic harms, especially physical and/or psychological damage to people. Prioritizing this seems simply to be another application of the oft-repeated injunction 'above all do no harm'. Even if other aspects of improvement are more controversial, it may seem comparably easy to justify the idea that health services shouldn't cause harms to patients. However, in practice, threshold priority lines are unlikely to be so clear-cut.

A distinction is sometimes drawn between those improvement activities which secure 'floors' and those which aspire towards 'ceilings'. The former would typically concentrate around ensuring that professional interventions are at least safe and sufficiently effective and the latter on more aspirational – and perhaps in some respects increasingly less 'central' and 'longer term' – aims and ideals relevant to offering the best care possible.[19] The idea of an improvement spectrum ranging from the 'must have' to the 'nice to have' may offer some guidance for improvement ethics, especially in relation to priority setting. It seems acceptable – and reflects the normal range of interests and commitments of healthcare practitioners – for improvers like Fatima to have and pursue a range of ambitions. Were her scope for improvement-related work more heavily circumscribed, however, it might be relevant for her to consider where on the 'must have' to 'nice to have' spectrum her various initiatives sit. She might judge that patient safety monitoring and the patient safety aspects of the clinical handover project are more urgent and should be her priority. One factor which comes into focus when time and resources for improvement are limited, and which might contribute to Fatima's decision, is the amount of risk improvers are willing to take. That is, there may be reason to prioritize the reduction of foreseeable preventable harms (even if relatively small) to known patients by demonstrated and reliable means over possible benefits (even if relatively large) to future patients by longer-term means with increased uncertainty about the efficacy of chosen approaches.

This is a plausible starting position. But the philosophical and ethical complications are extensive and suggest that this may not take us very far at all. Here we consider four reasons why operating with such a simple heuristic might be ill-advised. First, as discussed in Part 2, it is impossible to tidily disentangle separate dimensions of quality because they cluster together, interact and depend upon one another in many ways. Indeed, as we argued in Chapter 4, more recent ways of understanding and approaching the protection or promotion of safety (including Safety-II thinking) already problematize distinctions between safety and other quality dimensions such as effectiveness. Even to the extent that dimensions can be separated from one another, there are no decisive ways in which some are essential and others marginal. Organizing a service so that the avoidable harms it produces are substantially reduced is clearly a good thing. But so too, for example, is improving person-centredness and equity. Claims that an intervention reduces harms to 'a minimum' will be relatively uninformative about 'quality' unless they also specify whether the construction of 'minimum' includes or excludes the demands of other quality dimensions. (It would be possible to argue for a different and more inclusive sense of minimum here by suggesting that a proper conception and measure of safety would itself somehow incorporate other dimensions, but that would necessitate a lot of clarification and justification and is certainly not the way that 'safety' is understood by most improvers. In real-world, resource-constrained circumstances difficult questions about whether a less inclusive definition of harm is more appropriate would recur.)

Second, it is not necessarily the case that expertise related to short-term goals is especially applicable and reliable. Determining what is going to work, and how to make it work, in immediate specific contexts can itself be incredibly demanding. Furthermore, being able to 'put expertise to use' here and now will often depend upon much longer-term activities – such as approaches to initial and continuing education, helping to seed and grow a 'learning culture' within an organization and investment in research.[20]

Third, conceptions of purposes, standards and quality evolve over time. This means that something that is built into existing frameworks as a less pressing 'nice to have' might come to be judged retrospectively as an important but neglected priority. Examples here include proper respect and responsiveness in relation to aspects of personal identity, or levels of inclusion and personalization in decision-making, including particularly in agenda setting and not only picking from a prescribed 'choice menu'. These are things that have in recent history, and in many settings, come to be seen to matter a great deal but have previously been relatively neglected. In other words, improvers need to bear in mind both what we have called delivery and revisionary perspectives on improvement.

Finally, there are considerable philosophical uncertainties attached to balancing benefits to current patients and benefits to future patients. Many people will share an ethical intuition that favours attending to the visible needs of known people rather than the potential suffering of generalized abstract people in the future. This, for example, is why people demand that the victims of traffic accidents are properly tended to but may often show less interest in pressing for improvements in road safety policies and infrastructure that could prevent equivalently large (or greater) amounts of suffering and death in the future.[21] There are arguably independent reasons for caring about the patients in front of us – healthcare is, in part, about responsiveness to people with whom healthcare professionals have an existing relationship.[22] Not properly doing so feels, and some ethical accounts would argue is, different from indirectly letting down others. However, there is a genuine puzzle about when and how this 'privileging' of identifiable current patients over unknown future patients can be overdone. This is reflected in longstanding critical discussion of 'the rule of rescue' in relation to fair and sustainable healthcare resource allocation.[23] In highlighting this very important concern we do not want, as we have stressed already, to endorse the view that ethics simply involves a calculus of consequences and that any personal relational considerations should be seen as irrelevant. However, particularly in a universal or public healthcare system, there are undoubtedly reasons to make considerable space for longer-term and population-level policies, at the possible expense of shorter-term ones with direct and identifiable benefits.

This discussion of priorities connects to the distinction between 'delivery' and 'revisionary' perspectives on improvement. Improvement priorities are often delivery focused, that is, aiming to generate specific and relatively predictable improvements in relation to known and theoretically avoidable deficits. But more ambitious and radical improvements might aim to generate bigger and less predictable changes – such as an ambition to end race or gender discrimination in care, or to tackle healthcare recruitment and workforce crises. It can be extremely difficult to reason about how and whether to prioritize narrower but more certain and proximal benefits over wider, and potentially greater, but much less uncertain and more distant benefits. The risks associated with more transformative programmes of work can be difficult to justify in the short term, when compared with the lower hanging fruit of more delivery-focused improvements, but it is equally difficult to justify *not* tackling these bigger issues in the longer term, especially as they will also often beget delivery issues over time. Those setting improvement priorities must think about the balance between shorter and longer term, as well as more quotidian and more radical, improvement aims, as well as how these are liable to be interdependent, with action taken with respect to some aims affecting the possibility of pursuing other aims for better or for worse. While it might be tempting to assume that it is better to get the basics in place by tackling identified delivery gaps before tackling more complex and ambitious improvements, it is important to recognize that delays in tackling persistent systemic challenges have the potential to undermine improved delivery of services. And without consideration of their longer-term and wider implications, there is a risk that focusing on narrower and more proximal improvement efforts makes it more difficult to pursue more radical improvements.

In this section, we have discussed how prioritizing improvements requires consideration of different interpretations of 'urgency'. On the one hand, prioritization requires attention to how good or bad practice currently is in areas with the potential for improvement. On the other hand, we have suggested that there is reason to hesitate about prioritizing avoidance of more obvious or tangible harms over longer-term and less concrete improvement aspirations. This is most obvious when comparing a project that aims at short-term marginal and disputed safety gains with a longer-term project that may result in benefits for very many (including improvements in throughput and efficiency, or transformations in experiences of feeling cared for, which themselves may contribute substantially to patient safety). Nonetheless, there are risks attached to uncertain, aspirational and long-term improvement activities, and pursuing such activities may be judged imprudent when areas of healthcare remain inadequate or even dangerous, and there are plausible and well-evidenced ways of improving them. More generally, thinking about which 'bundles' of possible improvement activities to prioritize calls for a range of ways of thinking about priorities, including across conceptions and dimensions of quality, minimum and optimum standards, and shorter- and longer-term expectations and aspirations. There is no calculation that can tell improvers what to prioritize, nor a definitive list of factors to consider in making priority setting decisions; rather more deliberative and holistic ways of thinking are needed to support ethical decision-making in context.

6.4 Who does what (and how)?

Improvers don't only need to ask, '*what* should be done?' but '*who* should be doing what?' The task of identifying and pursuing improvement priorities is not performed by one exhaustively informed, boundlessly energetic and well-connected agent who does all the work: there are very many relevant agents and labour must be divided between them. This at least makes the possibility of tackling different kinds of tasks and agendas more feasible, although it also highlights the challenges of coordination and the potential for tensions and conflicts between the concerns of differently placed improvers.

The question of 'who should be doing what?' applies at two levels – first, in relation to improvement policies and practices and, second, in relation to caring responsibilities and roles. We will say something about both, but before doing so, it is worth underlining that the two levels are closely connected. Given that improvement is like public health and often seeks to reinforce, replace or inflect the expectations built into the contexts of healthcare, it might itself be seen to be about shaping the 'ethical landscape' of healthcare – by recommending, determining or encouraging specific allocations of caring responsibilities and roles and/ or by fostering specific kinds of cultures and dispositions.

The division of labour between improvers means that competing purposes can themselves be, to some extent, divided up. For example, some of the longer-term and revisionary improvement agendas might in the first instance be advanced by educators, regulators and policymakers, whereas some of the more pressing and 'remedial' delivery agendas need to sit with practitioners and managers closer to the ground. This is partly a function of what is possible for differently placed agents. Different healthcare actors have access to different kinds of 'levers'. In order to set or adjust targets or standards – at least those that are applied widely across institutions and systems – improvers will usually need to have the authority and social legitimacy that attaches to official professional governance or other forms of state-backed policymaking. But these relatively powerful actors cannot, at the same time, themselves deliver good practice on the ground. They can set parameters for practitioners and try to shape their conduct to some degree but, in practice, it is teams and individuals on the ground who need to define and deliver what matters.

This kind of division of labour is familiar from many working contexts including in healthcare. For example, clinicians are typically expected to do everything within their power to address patients' health problems, but they also work in contexts in which policymakers and regulators set limits on what medications and technologies are cost effective in order to manage population health and resources. The division between the 'on-the-ground' perspective and 'bird's-eye-view' perspective is not just pragmatic in the sense that not everyone can do everything all at once, but also necessary to preserve possibilities and forms of professionalism. If clinicians on the ground were constantly reimagining healthcare and solely thinking in revisionary terms about improvement, they wouldn't be able to fulfil some of their core professional duties of caring for patients in line with currently understood and available best practice. Obviously the activities of different agents need to somehow 'join up' and this requires people to take account of one another's agendas. Another way of putting this is to say that there is no single hierarchy of priorities but multiple hierarchies reflecting different vantage points. This means that a lack of cohesion – and tensions of various kinds – should not be seen wholly as a sign of disorganization. Tensions between competing improvement agendas can be seen as necessary and even valuable insofar as they are acknowledged and help different parties be mindful about different perspectives and goals.

It seems sensible to take the prevailing healthcare division of labour seriously when discussing the distribution of responsibilities. One relevant starting point is 'What am I supposed to be doing?' This helps to cut through any suggestion that an improvement agenda is wholly open-ended because, in principle, improvers could 'start from anywhere'. For example, Fatima is a paediatric consultant and it makes sense to assume that she should start by focusing on the needs of her working context and making use of the levers that are relatively close to hand. But the need for some division of labour in improvement should not set strict limits to the ambitions of specific practitioners. Improvers should be wary of assuming that the norms and priorities embedded in current settings exhaust the parameters around which improvement agendas should be developed. On the account we gave above, Fatima is committed to broad-ranging and ambitious rethinking of the nature of professional roles and norms and is engaged in collective working to advance these at a more structural level. Healthcare improvement looks beyond the immediate provision of care towards shaping that provision, so citing existing 'role expectations' will not be decisive. This is in many respects comparable to the case of clinical ethics: clinicians are expected to do their jobs and, at least sometimes, to be able to stand back from them and be ready to question the way their working context is defined. But placing weight on existing parameters becomes even more problematic to the extent that what we are seeking to do is precisely to question and improve things. When someone puts on an improvement hat, their role becomes, to some degree, more analogous to that of rule-maker than a rule-follower.

Improvers need, therefore, to be conscious that they are changing the 'ethical landscape' for other people. This is an important facet of the normative consciousness we are calling for. As was reflected in the discussion of public health, one of the functions of improvement interventions is to change the way other agents think and act (just as no smoking policies change the norms and activities of workers in shops, libraries or restaurants). Improvement involves trying to reinforce or change norms and expectations, which results in intended and unintended effects for services, staff and patients. Improvement interventions may, for example, seek to create new sets of responsibilities and foster certain kinds of dispositions. In relation to the effects on health professionals, this should entail some careful ethical reflection amongst improvers: are the forms of influence used – including the degree of compulsion, encouragement, voluntariness adopted – not only potentially effective but also justifiable? Do they treat other people with sufficient respect and fairly? And what are some of the possible 'side effects' of the proposed change? (For example, a diminution in professional discretion may increase reliability in some respects but may also reduce flexibility, responsiveness, motivation and individual accountability.)

The possible effects are broader than influence over professional roles and the division of labour within formal health services. For instance, all those improvement policies that aim (often for very good reason) to move treatments, care and patient monitoring away from hospital and towards community and home settings are – directly or indirectly – creating new responsibilities for families and other carers, and for people to 'self-manage'. Both the vocational benefits and burdens of caring are being, to some degree, reallocated and this raises questions, for example, about capacity and lines of accountability. How far this is a good thing will surely vary from case to case but there is no doubt that it is ethically significant and requires consideration rather than skating over.

Anyone engaging in healthcare improvement finds themselves in a complex, multi-layered ethical landscape that are navigating and, to some extent, shaping. Ideally, they will be mindful about other people's agendas and ready to consciously manage the tensions between what they judge to be better and various kinds of 'official expectations', including the tensions between competing improvement agendas.

One crucial and easily neglected consideration is the more diffuse 'constitutive' effect of improvement. The aim of improvement is to change the world, but improvement activities are also part of the world.

This should be obvious but can be obscured. There is a danger that improvement interventions can be treated as parallel mechanisms and 'bracketed out' as if they were 'shadow activities' like those of backstage staff at the theatre, not part of the dramatic action. This is another reason why asking whether or not improvement interventions produce the desired results is insufficient. Improvers must also ask whether the ways in which improvement is enacted make the world better and are ethically acceptable or ideal. This is true for specific improvement interventions but especially for the cumulative effects of improvement structures and cultures. Within a health system, or within a single institution, does the way in which improvement is conceived, organized, funded and practised have negative (as well as positive) effects? In addition to highlighting the resource costs and risks of efforts going wrong this brings back into view several concerns raised earlier in this chapter and the book. One central question here is about the cumulative effects of the ways in which improvement structures and cultures frame 'better healthcare', for example, the unanticipated effects of putting a strong emphasis on specific forms of measurement or of monitoring and measuring some things and not others.[24]

6.5 Moving from technical to expansive ways of thinking

Bringing ethics into healthcare improvement research and practice calls for diffuse forms of attention. Improvement ethics means looking at improvement interventions in a range of contexts. This includes seeing them as part of a wider process of asking questions about what counts as making things better, seeing interventions not solely in isolation but as part of a policy mix that includes many shared improvement efforts, and as occurring within systems and social fields that themselves require ethical discussion and debate. There are underlying questions about what the purposes of improvement ought to be and what vision of healthcare underpins healthcare improvement. This links with questions about relative priorities that include striking the right balances between delivery and revisionary perspectives and between securing quality 'floors' and being more aspirational, even idealistic. The result is that there is not only one set of ethical questions here – is the end goal reached and is the method acceptable? – but many intersecting layers of questions and uncertainties.

Moving away from purely technical thinking necessitates confronting the ways in which means and ends cannot be neatly separated out. To practise improvement is not to exercise neutral, frictionless levers. What we have called 'forms of influence' need ethical investigation as do the ways improvement activities embody values. To take an obvious example, if an improvement activity seeks to improve communication and trust amongst stakeholders in a service, it would be strange and concerning for those steering it to use methods that don't including listening and respect. It is not simply that disrespectful methods are unlikely to work but that, by definition, they undermine what is being pursued.

Improvement activities do not sit outside healthcare realities, they help constitute and create those realities. Improvers need to be ready to ask whether they embody or reinforce systems and cultures that are damaging, for example, because of their unintended macro-effects or because of institutional sexism, racism or less clear-cut forms of discrimination or insensitivity. Tackling or inadvertently reinforcing forms of exclusion is one of the ways that improvement may impact on the 'ethical landscape' of healthcare. Generally, improvers need to be mindful of the way improvement activity works (and sometimes is designed) to inflect and reshape ethics, for example, by creating new aims or goals, new obligations, and encouraging or discouraging certain dispositions.

We suggest that opening up this range of complexity in improvement ethics is one of the products of understanding that improvement happens within complex social systems. As discussed in Chapter 2, we see the idea of 'normative complexity' as analogous to, and overlapping with, the idea of 'explanatory complexity' that is already recognized within the field of improvement by those with an interest in complex, adaptive systems. Normative complexity is a product of many factors. In Part 2 we discussed and illustrated how it stems from the ways in which what counts as good healthcare is contested – involving a combination of multiple dimensions, interpretations and perspectives. We have just been discussing how it also reflects the ways in which improving healthcare entails thinking and acting across bundles of intersecting policies and practices, numerous relevant roles and responsibilities, and possible effects at macro- and micro-levels and over shorter- and longer-term timescales. Normative complexity parallels, and interacts with, explanatory complexity. Just as it is a mistake to conceive of improvement interventions as taking place along single causal lines when they are entangled within multiple intersecting lines and contexts, it is a mistake to think of ethics appraisal as something that can take place simply by looking at single interventions in isolation or by applying any one tidy evaluative framework. Ethical appraisal involves taking into account something analogous to the 'feedback loops' that are discussed in the context of explanatory complexity. The prima facie desirable effects of an intervention may be reinforced or cancelled out by other effects (e.g. on other dimensions of quality, or for different communities, etc.) not just causally but, in addition, in terms of how they can be positively or negatively evaluated when judged in combination and/or from more revisionary standpoints. Embracing the open-endedness of improvement ethics demands holistic, imaginative and dialogical ways of thinking.

This review of the scope of the field suggests that the ethics of healthcare improvement might be seen as an intellectual and practical quagmire. That it is not only a hazardous area but one that it is impossible to navigate. That is a legitimate worry, not least because this perception may have the effect of putting people off the subject. We definitely do not want to encourage this and that is why the next chapter considers potential navigation aids.

7 PRACTISING IMPROVEMENT

In this chapter we argue that giving a higher profile to ethical issues in healthcare improvement, and in particular building cultures and practices that address them, can substantially strengthen the field. Here there is a parallel with the clinical work of medical, nursing and other healthcare professionals. Clinical professionalism is shaped not only by an ethical orientation but by conscious attention to the ethical dimension of clinical care. An account of clinical professionalism that omitted this dimension would be seriously distorted and dangerous. Given that improvement work is designed to affect professional practices and the health outcomes and experiences of many people, the same assumption should apply. The parallel can be extended further. It would be a mistake to think of ethics as an alien material that has been grafted onto clinical professionalism; rather it is in large measure inherent in and integrated within it. There is a place for 'external voices' – from patient groups and from academics such as philosophers – to challenge the prevailing assumptions and norms of clinical work. But these voices need to make sense to, and be in (sometimes critical) dialogue with, professional communities who already 'speak ethics'.

In earlier chapters (starting in Chapter 2) we have talked about the ways in which ethics is effectively 'built into' improvement work. This chapter starts by further unpacking and elaborating on this idea. We highlight some of the perspectives on and approaches to ethics that are already to some degree embedded in healthcare improvement. We suggest that these provide a substantial basis for improvement ethics, and one that can and should be developed. We look, in turn, at four broad kinds of expectations and practices that have some presence in the field and that can contribute to the management of ethical complexity:

1 expectations and practices of accountability;

2 the recognition and cultivation of 'good habits' in improvement;

3 an emphasis on, and the valuing of, listening and conversation; and

4 engagement with contributions from bioethics or applied philosophy.

These are four discrete and contrasting 'starting points' for a discussion about ethics but here we suggest, more boldly, that these practices provide a foundation for – and in important respects *are* – improvement ethics – albeit a version of improvement ethics that needs to be extended and enriched. In particular, we suggest that improvement ethics should become more self-conscious, in some respects more systematic, as well as more recognized and collectively supported within professional and policy cultures. Later in the chapter we also argue for improvement ethics to be more far reaching and open-ended in scope. Healthcare improvement would benefit from greater ethical challenge, including from external voices. Existing practices are valuable and necessary but, unless they can extend to embrace critical challenge, are insufficient.

In what follows we discuss the relevance and potential implications of these four interconnected sets of practices. In so doing, we hope to illuminate the complementarities between them. Some of these are hopefully obvious – for instance, ethics rests upon good habits amongst which expectations around dialogic working are a prominent feature, with accountability practices being one important example. In the course of the chapter, we sketch out an increasingly holistic picture of improvement ethics. In particular, we move away from any assumption that ethics is primarily about 'big decision points' and authoritative 'stamps of approval', and towards an account in which the negotiation of ethical issues is more pervasive and includes the many ways in which improvers sensitize themselves to and make sense of what is ethically salient in their working environments and practices, including by routinely talking and listening to others. In unpacking these issues, we also indicate some possible tensions between our four themes, depending on how they are interpreted. For example, in concluding, we note the potential for applied philosophy to raise questions that are not bounded by the imperatives of day-to-day practice, and to look beyond prevailing conceptions of improvement – the agenda for Part 4 of this book. This chapter, taken as a whole, seeks to show both that healthcare improvement has its own existing resources for handling ethics and that these resources would benefit from more engagement with philosophical questioning and perspectives.

7.1 Building accountability

It is a standard expectation that those undertaking improvements will be in a position to 'give some account' of themselves – at least to be able to explain what they are aiming to do, how they have gone about it and why they think it matters. This is largely taken for granted and, as a result, may not be routinely highlighted, but it is central to ethics. The giving of some account is unavoidable if only for the pragmatic reason that improvement actors will be asking things of other people and will have to make their plans seem both intelligible and defensible to them. Although such an account may sometimes be cast largely in scientific terms, it might also be said, in an ethical idiom, that improvers 'owe' others this account. Furthermore, given the fact that improvement involves 'interference' in people's work and lives, accountability can be assumed to involve some element of ethical justification.

Providing a very explicit and systematic description of an intervention – including the assumptions underlying it, processes of reasoning followed, context and practices of intervention – is a core constitutive feature of scientific study. It makes it possible for other researchers to 'check', or critically examine, the scientific basis of interventions and, within limits and taking into account context variations, to 'replicate' the same kind of work, thereby reinforcing or amending the evidence base. This kind of relatively exact 're-calculating' conception of accountability can only be applied to technically defined and circumscribed actions, but something closely analogous has a much broader relevance. Accountability in this broader sense involves 'the procedures and processes by which one party justifies and takes responsibility for its activities',[1] and the idea of 'replicability' can still be seen as relevant although in a more elastic form. As Albert Weale puts it in his discussion of replicability and accountability in public life beyond science:

> Given the inherent plurality entailed by human reasoning, we should not expect any particular piece of reasoning to secure widespread consensus. Different individuals may still follow the train of reasoning,

without agreeing on it. What is necessary is that they should be able to follow it as a train of reasoning. That is, they ought to be able to say: given those premises and that body of evidence, I can see how someone might come to this conclusion (even though it is not necessarily the conclusion I would come to myself).[2]

While some form of transparency is needed for accountability, more is required. As suggested in the accounts above, accountability requires the accountable party to inform others about and provide justification for their actions. It is also typically taken to involve an accounting party with the capacity to pass judgements and perhaps impose sanctions or other consequences – that is, there is someone or some organization to whom those accounting are accountable.[3] While contemporary invocations of accountability in relation to public institutions tend to demand or assume that this involves public scrutiny, accountability does not necessarily require public broadcast, just reporting to the accounting party.

Within the relatively limited literature on the ethics of healthcare improvement, the need for, and potential demands of accountability have been most thoroughly discussed in relation to the institutional governance of proposed improvement interventions. In 2003, the Hastings Center convened a substantial project on the governance of improvement ethics which brought together experts from healthcare improvement and bioethics.[4] The project group suggested a framework for understanding and approaching ethical accountability in improvement work. Whilst, of course, this framework can be subjected to critique it provides a very helpful basis for thinking about the relevant issues.[5] The key idea advanced is that improvement activities rest on reciprocal ethical requirements. That is, under normal circumstances, clinicians, managers and patients have duties to accept, and where necessary participate in, improvement interventions (and activities necessary to plan or monitor them) so long as these interventions themselves meet a range of ethical requirements.

The Hastings Center project focused on 'quality improvement' (QI) as one construction of healthcare improvement. It defines QI as 'systematic, data-guided activities designed to bring about immediate improvements in health care delivery in particular settings'.[6] Given this account, the project group conclude that QI is an intrinsic part of normal healthcare and good clinical practice. In other words, healthcare professionals are somehow duty bound by their roles to engage with and participate in healthcare improvement. However, of course it does not follow that they are thereby bound to engage in improvement activities uncritically. Improvement ethics demands a certain level of critical analysis in the development and enactment of improvement activities. This does not mean everyone has to critically analyse all the time, but it does require some meaningful assurance that interventions and projects have been subject to appropriately rigorous ethical scrutiny.

The framework's authors set out what they called ethical requirements for the conduct of improvement interventions and recommendations for implementing accountability for such conduct. Both indicate valuable directions for developing improvement ethics. We briefly summarize some of the requirements here, although our main interest here is less in the details and more in reflecting on the aspiration the project represents.

The ethical requirements fall into seven topics or themes:

1 *Social or scientific value* – that the gains sought justify the resources used and risks to participants;

2 *Scientific validity* – that the approach should be methodologically sound;

3 *Fair participant selection* – selection aimed at a 'fair distribution of burdens and benefits of QI';

4 *Favourable risk–benefit ratio* – the design of QI activity should limit risks and maximize benefits, and risks to individual participants should be balanced by benefits to them where possible;

5 *Respect for participants* – covers a range of considerations including protecting privacy and confidentiality, information provision about the improvement intervention and its results, sharing results with wider health system in ways which don't identify individuals (without their consent);

6 *Informed consent* – where there is minimal risk, this is to be assumed within patient consent to treatment; with greater risk then specific consent for QI activities should be sought. Risk for patients or staff should be measured relative to the usual risks of undergoing or providing standard healthcare;

7 *Independent review* – ethical review should be proportionate to the level of risks. In many cases this means that accountability for QI should be seen as integrated within accountability for clinical care. In some cases QI should face a review that is more comparable to (or integrated with) ethical review of research projects.[7]

An important conclusion of this project is that, for the most part, accountability for improvement should not be 'exported' into systems for reviewing research ethics but rather 'ethical oversight of QI should become part of an enhanced accountability system for professional responsibility and the supervision and management of clinical care'.[8] It is worth underlining that the call here is for 'an enhanced accountability system'. That is, there is no presumption that whatever systems of clinical accountability are in place are already adequate for overseeing improvement activities (nor perhaps, indeed, clinical activities). But the emphasis is on establishing that improvement projects are part of 'normal work' and in that regard, in most cases, unlike research. (The authors take care to articulate the criteria that indicate which improvement projects also count as research and should be subject to research oversight.)[9] We discussed the question of the analogies and disanalogies between improvement and research in Chapter 6 and it is a subject that other authors have debated, sometimes coming to different conclusions.[10] It is not a debate that we wish to dwell upon further here, but we do want to highlight one of the key issues that lies behind it: the question of 'burdensomeness'.

The line the Hastings Center project group take is founded on the recognition that ethical review processes are not themselves cost-free. Any review process that is, in their terms, relatively 'costly' and 'cumbersome' would constitute, on their account, an obstacle to necessary improvements. It would 'mean that managers would have reason to make changes without monitoring effects or to leave malfunctioning care arrangements unchanged'.[11] Just as improvement activities do not 'float above' ethics in some neutral frictionless zone, neither do ethical review activities. In assessing the balance the project team aimed to strike, it is important to reinforce the point that here they have in mind improvement activities that are relatively low-risk, small-scale, incremental, data-led and carefully monitored. Insofar as activities depart from this assumption different approaches are needed.

Assuming that this is a sound, or at least plausible, argument against excessive degrees of formal institutional oversight, a very significant challenge remains. Granted that there might be good reason for improvers to reduce levels of practical and bureaucratic burdensomeness, how should they treat the additional cognitive, personal and social burdensomeness of ethical accountability? Being able to 'give an account' in relation to an improvement project means that those responsible should (at least in principle) be able not only to set out the technical basis for the project but also to have adequate responses to questions about how the project fulfils the 'ethical requirements' summarized above. Similarly there should be some potential for such responses to be, at minimum, open to scrutiny or discussion at an institutional level. On the one hand, it seems wholly plausible that would-be improvers, including those undertaking small-scale and closely monitored interventions, should be required to consider, and account for, the ethical defensibility of their initiatives. On the other hand, there seems to be a genuine worry about how demanding this requirement should be if it is to be feasible in practice and not dismissed as unrealistic. Can ethical accountability be made practical?

In the framework, ethical accountability entails, 'Health care professionals and organizations need a robust understanding of the ethical requirements for QI, and organizations must have procedures to ensure that QI activities meet ethical standards.'[12] We briefly consider each of these things – 'robust understanding' and 'procedures' – in relation to the question of burdensomeness.

Turning first to the need for 'robust understanding': the seven 'ethical requirements' listed above can easily be interpreted in ways that makes understanding their implications cognitively burdensome for all concerned. The first four requirements alone necessitate that improvers are satisfied that overall benefits outweigh risks, that burdens and benefits are distributed fairly, and that the chosen approach is methodologically robust. Given the contentiousness – including the levels of explanatory and normative complexity – explored in the previous chapters, meeting these requirements adequately presents a highly demanding intellectual agenda, and may arguably even pose inherently unresolvable puzzles. The same level of intellectual burden – again leaving aside any question about formal institutional mechanisms – would seem to apply to anyone scrutinizing possible responses to these requirements.

Development and use of appropriate 'procedures' could help to contain (rather than intensify) concerns about burdensomeness. Well-designed procedures can, in theory at least, bestow ethical legitimacy while also to some extent managing uncertainty by setting out expectations regarding what is required in terms of 'understanding'. The well-recognized burdens of ethical review processes – in terms of time, paperwork, institutional and professional accommodations and negotiations and so on – carry the advantage that clearly visible and well-documented processes have been defined, for example. Although such processes can be frustrating and sometimes seem to either over-govern or be insufficiently sensitive, or both, those on either side of them have a good idea of what is expected.

The recommendations of the Hastings Center project group point in a different direction from the more formal accountability associated with ethical review.[13] The central suggestion that accountability for (routine) improvement should be integrated into professional supervision of clinical practice neither assumes existing supervision is adequate nor places reliance on some extra or external mechanism. The tenor of the recommendations is holistic and the authors encourage exploration and evolution rather than specified fixes or formal standards. Recommendations include: building literacy about improvement and related responsibilities and ethics within professional organizations, accrediting bodies and healthcare institutions; patient education about rights and responsibilities; and the strengthening of methodological expertise and guidance for improvement practices including in relation to ethics. The institutional 'internal management' of improvement activities is only one element identified and here the recommendation is that 'arrangements for internal management ... should be translated into models that will work in real health care settings'.[14] This includes, for those improvement activities that meet the threshold for research, potentially adapting research governance arrangements so they are suited for improvement-related research projects, and trialling and gaining experience in such adaptations. While instructive, these recommendations are relatively light on the detail of what legitimate procedures must look like in order to secure ethical accountability.

We suggest two somewhat exaggerated but broadly plausible ways of interpreting the implications of the project group's work on ethical accountability. On the one hand, the 'ethical requirements' can be interpreted as a kind of stiff intellectual examination. This might be compared to someone planning a healthcare improvement being given an examination paper and asked to demonstrate how their proposal meets specified criteria of ethical acceptability. On the other hand, the 'implementing accountability recommendations' can be interpreted in much more distributed and collegial terms – they call for system-wide evolutionary change that helps build shared literacy about improvement ethics and creates enlarged expectations about ethical reflection and dialogue.

There is a way of reading these two interpretations as convergent but for now we choose to highlight contrasts. The first – 'examination' – interpretation has the potential to be extremely severe. Even taking one ethical requirement – say, fair distribution of benefits and burdens – there are (as set out in Chapter 5) multiple interpretations of what this idea might mean and entail in practice and such interpretations are inherently contestable. And this is supposing that an examiner is happy to live with the idea that improvement interventions can be considered singly and defended on their own terms, and do not require more synoptic and systemic assessment. But arguments rehearsed earlier, including in Chapter 6, suggest that a simple focus on discrete interventions does not suffice. That is, that ethical analysis should include questioning the underlying rationale and purposes of improvement efforts and not just their approach, and it should also look at their combined and cumulative effects, including 'landscape shaping' effects, on systems and cultures. Our earlier analyses suggest there are grounds for saying the Hastings Center group's recommendations are rather narrowly drawn. For example, as well as paying attention to and respecting 'participants', such as current patients, recommendations could reasonably ask for account to be taken of the interests and perspectives of a much wider range of stakeholders – including all those individuals, communities and agencies who are implicated in, or affected by, changes to healthcare institutions, including future citizens and patients. In short, given a rigorous examiner it would be extremely difficult to pass the examination.

The second – 'collegial' – interpretation could be seen as gentler and less exacting although, at the same time, as offering less definitive verdicts on whether criteria have been met and who should be held accountable. It involves wide-ranging learning processes through which thinking about and discussing improvement ethics become steadily more commonplace. The burdens and practices of accountability are shared out and individual improvers become sensitized, and more accustomed, to reflecting on a range of potential ethical complications. This collegial interpretation remains in danger of falling short of meaningful accountability, however, to the extent that the forms of justification it involves are diverse and informal, and there is no clear party to whom improvers are accountable.

In practice, familiar versions of ethical accountability in healthcare sit somewhere between these two conceptions. Researchers facing ethics committees are confronted with something like an official examination but the pass mark is not set to make a judgement about whether all possible ethical issues, seen from every critical angle, have been fully addressed. The challenge is not to prove that the proposed research will be ethically impeccable, but rather to show that a subset of conspicuous ethical risks have been acknowledged and will be carefully managed. For the most part, clinical ethics conforms more to the second conception of accountability: there is no official 'exam' but the background assumption is that clinicians will have developed practical experience and insight into the ethical dimensions of their work and will be surrounded by similarly experienced colleagues who offer their own perspective and counsel where that is needed. There are likely to be investigatory and disciplinary procedures in place for grossly negligent and dangerous practice, but these are used in exceptional cases, and the forms of accountability governing quotidian practice are more collegial. This is the background against which the Hastings Center project group recommend that much of improvement ethics should be seen as more like clinical than research forms of ethical accountability. There are also hybrid models – a useful comparator is the 'minimal risk' ethics procedures that apply in some places, in which researchers who have become accustomed to addressing research ethics are encouraged to have reflected on, and take responsibility for, the ethics of a proposed project and, as a result, face very limited external scrutiny.

The focus of the next section of this chapter overlaps with the more collegial conception of accountability which, we suggest, reflects a valuable perspective on professional ethics. However, we also think there is a place for the first conception in which ethics is seen as posing probing, demanding, and as a result sometimes destabilizing questions. Later in the chapter – when we consider how philosophy might contribute to improvement ethics – we return to this more demanding conception.

7.2 Cultivating good habits

There is no need to continuously question the motivations of improvers (although later we flag up circumstances in which one might). Indeed, as we noted before, it seems reasonable to describe their motivations in ethical terms: reducing the risks of healthcare and improving patient outcomes and experiences are ethically important matters. The same is, of course, true of those aims that are more overtly value-oriented – for example, being concerned that healthcare is equitable or person-centred. In addition, there are a range of ethically relevant qualities that are encouraged within the improvement field. It is, for example, normal for improvers to be expected to approach their work conscientiously, to be explicit about their aims and methods, and to closely monitor and report the effects of their interventions. As discussed in Section 7.1, these expectations are among the key planks of ethical accountability.

In large areas of our lives, and arguably most of the time, ethics is not treated as primarily an intellectual activity. This applies, for example, to the way people make ethical appraisals of friends and colleagues – in relation to people's actions, inclinations and attitudes rather than simply by an analysis of their ethical reasoning. Virtue theory is one branch of ethical theory that emphasizes this more holistic, 'whole person' way of conceptualizing ethics. People's 'virtues' are their admirable habitual dispositions – such as their conscientiousness, honesty and kindness.[15] Virtue theory emphasizes questions about people's commitments, motivations and character and reduces the centrality of abstract questions about formulating and resolving ethical dilemmas. From this perspective, experience, good habits and 'practical wisdom' (which we elaborate on shortly) make up the basis and engine of ethics. Virtues are human attributes that are characteristically linked to particular practices, and which enable those who possess them to achieve the goods internal to those practices.[16] They are widely invoked in the context of professional ethics because they are sensitive to the contextual ethical features and challenges which characterize different professions, roles and workplaces, and the way that professional identities can be collegially constructed and maintained.[17] While there may be difficult judgement calls to be made about right and wrong professional action, a virtue-focused conception of professional identity will stress that when such calls arise, they should be met by a workforce of colleagues who have developed a relevant 'track record' such that, ideally, they have become ethically discriminating and adroit.

Thinking about the development of improvement ethics from this angle emphasizes not only the dispositions of individuals but also the structural and cultural conditions in which improvement (and healthcare) activities operate. This includes, for example, the kinds of education and in-service training and development in place to underpin improvement work. How far do working conditions and professional development support ethical awareness and 'good habits?' In response to this question, we suggest that there is quite a lot to be positive about, as well as, of course, more that could be done. We start by identifying how habits might be seen as building blocks in a 'professional ethics' of improvement, including some of the 'good habit-supporting' currents and tendencies in the field. But, in concluding this section, we acknowledge the risks of too great a reliance on this way of thinking.

Bill Lucas, drawing on work with Hadjer Nacer and research and exchanges with groups of experienced improvement practitioners and academics, presents a broad overview of what are described as the 'habits of an improver'.[18] These are the good habits that are, or at least should be, cultivated by induction into a community of healthcare improvement, either as a specialist or as a health professional committed to improvement. There is a sense in which these habits constitute healthcare improvement identities and practices: 'Spend any time with someone for whom improvement is an intrinsic part of their job and you realize that they think and act in different ways from those who are simply set on routine service delivery.'[19] Lucas and Nacer describe five habits that underpin a conscientious and effective orientation to improvement: *learning, influencing, resilience, creativity* and *systems thinking*. Their account draws on, and makes analogies with, a previous study of the 'real-world learning' of professional engineers.

An important component of their argument – central to our interests here – is that professional capabilities are too often discussed in overly narrow terms. In particular, there is a tendency in constructing curricula to foreground 'knowledge' and 'skills'. Whilst these aspects of learning are clearly necessary, they are, in a fundamental way, insufficient. It is not only that having knowledge and skills is compatible with failing to put them into practice, but also that one might be said not to have fully learned and developed knowledge and skills except to the extent that one has consistently practised them, in a variety of circumstances over time, and has come to do so as a matter of habit. Lucas and Nacer unpack their five habits into fifteen sub-habits:[20]

1 *Learning*: questioning, problem finding, reflective;

2 *Influencing*: empathetic, facilitative, comfortable with conflict;

3 *Resilience*: optimistic, calculated risk taking, tolerating uncertainty;

4 *Creativity*: generating ideas, critical thinking, team playing;

5 *Systems thinking*: connection making, synthesizing, accepting change.

We are not going to discuss their account in depth or try to assess its merits, but the underlying thrust of this approach is an important one. In summary it is that something like 'improvement professionalism' is underpinned by achieving what in 'human resource' contexts is now often called the correct 'person specification' and 'personal qualities'.

Lucas and Nacer locate their account against the psychology and professional learning literatures but there are strong parallels, and some overlap with, a virtue theory approach to ethics. Embodied expertise and dispositions are central to professional ethics. A world in which every decision had to be thought through from first principles would be one characterized by inertia and ineptitude. The fifteen sub-habits make no explicit reference to ethics and could, we suggest, be extended and elaborated in ways that capture the kinds of ethical sensitivities and discriminations needed within improvement work, but they are already directly relevant to improvement ethics. First, if the motivations of improvement are broadly ethical ones, then the capabilities that enable people to accomplish them are ethically important. Second, some of the listed habits and sub-habits highlight the extent to which the core capabilities required are about 'right relations' with other people – for example, being empathic and facilitative, being able to work with others, make connections between people and handle the conflicts this gives rise to. It is worth briefly reiterating that these kinds of capabilities, which the work on improvement habits and the range of expert voices that fed into it see as central to improvement practice, indicate that the field of improvement extends beyond merely 'technical' activity.

The improvement habits paper, although it does not feature the language of virtues, cites the Ancient Greek, and particularly Aristotelian, idea of 'phronesis' (or 'practical wisdom') as a relevant comparator for, or even description of, the approach adopted. Practical wisdom is a central notion within the tradition of virtue ethics and has also been cited as important in other work on healthcare improvement practice and research.[21] At its most general, the idea indicates something like experience-based and context-responsive practical judgement, and it is contrasted with more logical and theoretical forms of knowledge. In this general sense, practical wisdom is relevant to what is sometimes construed as a theory-practice gap in professional work. When operating in real-world settings abstract knowledge can inform practice but cannot be 'directly' applied to it; rather, applied knowledge has to be constructed around and respond to the practical circumstances that prevail. The more specific sense of practical wisdom, as used and explained within virtue ethics, is closely related to this general idea; indeed, it refers, roughly speaking, to what is involved in possessing and exercising the experience-based forms of insight and deliberation that make up 'ethical knowledge' in practice.[22]

Being ethical arguably involves a combination of knowledge and practical wisdom. Someone might assess the ethical judgement and integrity of a colleague by looking at the evidence of their actions, feelings and desires as much as by the assertions they make about what is ethically correct. To say that someone is fair, for example, is to capture something about who they are and how they act, and consistently so, and not just their ability to answer questions about fairness fluently. But, of course, cognitive elements play an important role. In virtue ethics the business of ethical development is seen as something that is cultivated over time by practice – people learn to be fair not just by learning relevant concepts but by practising fairness in the ways they act, such that it becomes 'second nature'. There is a big gap, however, between saying that something is second nature and saying it is wholly automatic like a 'knee jerk'. Sometimes knowing what is called for will be relatively simple and spontaneous – if you are, for example, cutting up a cake to share with friends your default 'unthinking' tendency will be to try to divide it into same-sized portions. Often, however, what is called for will not be obvious but will require knowledge and understanding, including being responsive to circumstances and balancing multiple case-specific considerations together. What is cultivated over time by practice – including critical reflection where needed – is not just habit but the practical wisdom to apply and adapt habits by being sensitive to situations and their varying, and sometimes unique, demands. Virtuous conduct is not simply about having general dispositions such as honesty, kindness or fairness – dispositions that can pull in different directions – but consists in the developed capacity to combine and orchestrate these together into activity that meets the needs of specific circumstances.

We suggest that this kind of approach to ethics – ethics seen as embodied experience, discernment and practical navigation – has a good deal to contribute to improvement ethics. As signalled earlier, we also suggest that it provides a more encouraging and positive account of the resources available for developing and strengthening improvement ethics than one based mainly on 'add-on' intellectual analysis. In much of the remainder of this section and the next one we illustrate this positive account. Our illustration includes highlighting some 'models and mechanisms' within existing improvement approaches that support practical wisdom. But, in the conclusion to this section, we stress some of the limitations of reliance on these models and mechanisms, and more broadly the need to complement an emphasis on good habits and practical judgement with a more philosophically analytic approach to ethics.

The discussion of epistemic humility in Chapter 5 represents both a valuable example and an important theme for our positive account. Epistemic humility is a key virtue for those practising healthcare improvement. At the same time as recognizing that there is often an ethical imperative to improve healthcare (most clearly where services fall short of recognized standards and cause harm through action or omission), it is essential that improvers also seriously question their own knowledge base and contributions. Even granted that something is wrong in a particular instance, how can they be confident that their actions are making things better and not worse? As mentioned in Chapter 5, one of the mechanisms that can support epistemic humility is the use of multiple measures. Instead of relying on one or two simple measures to show the effects of an intervention (e.g. showing that 'throughput' has increased and 'safety incidents' decreased) potential changes can usefully be considered from multiple angles (e.g. in addition to these factors, are some subgroup of patients relatively disadvantaged by the change, is the change sustainable in terms of professional workload, does the improvement intervention produce complications for or shortcomings in other parts of a service or system?).

This example is illustrative in both theoretical and substantive ways. At a theoretical level it shows how virtues and practical judgement can be encouraged and supported by cultures and social practices. It is much harder for an individual practitioner to exercise epistemic humility in a context where this is relatively anomalous or exceptional, than where it is expected, encouraged and even incentivized. The latter climate will also, as a result, be one in which this virtue is more likely to be cultivated and reinforced. Fortunately, the expectation that multiple measures are important is built into many approaches to healthcare improvement, for example, the highly influential 'Model for Improvement' calls for the use of 'balancing measures' to ensure practitioners look beyond their target concern.[23] In practice, however, the balancing measures that will enable a holistic assessment of the impact of improvement interventions may be difficult for improvers to capture; localized and small-scale improvement projects are unlikely, for example, to be able to measure the impact of changes on other parts of the healthcare system or to track long-term outcomes.

At the level of substance, the need for multiple measures is just one indication of the level of complexity attached to both planning and evaluating improvement activities. In relation to the levels of normative complexity we have discussed, more is needed by way of response than the use of multiple measures. Those working on improvement and considering claims about quality also need to acknowledge that measures are inherently partial and should be treated with a degree of scepticism. This much is required simply to help underpin and practise epistemic humility, and it provides a small indication of what might be involved in offering a full account of the capabilities needed for practical wisdom in healthcare improvement (along the lines attempted in the 'habits of an improver' paper). The related case for 'skeptical calculative cultures' as advanced by Pflueger,[24] and introduced in Chapter 5, reflects not only the fact that characterizations of quality are multidimensional but also that measures reflect different standpoints and concerns. Measures are not neutral descriptions of 'what is there'; rather they 'make up', or are constitutive of, our conceptions of quality and, as we have underlined, they are shaped by particular purposes and perspectives and have a range of effects. Once this is recognized, Pflueger argues, improvers must abandon any presumption that a single true and precise account can be achieved by aiming for unified, standardized and centralized measures, and recognize that 'truth' and precision are better achieved by consciously working with 'incomplete', 'messy', 'overlapping' and 'conflicting' accounts. Here practical wisdom precludes placing undue weight on reductionist stories. We echo Pflueger's suggestion that this does not undermine the possibility of accountability to others but, as discussed in Section 7.1, shows how improvers might work with a richer, and thus more credible, notion of what accountability entails.

There are a range of practical supports to practical wisdom, including epistemic humility, within the healthcare improvement field. In addition to the in-built recognition that quality is multidimensional and calls for multiple measures, there are currents that reflect and encourage attention to complexity. These include the valuing of qualitative data and methods, 'soft intelligence' and 'stakeholder' voices.

Together these things help to capture the messiness of the social world, the inherently interpretive component of our readings of it, and the existence of multiple vantage points and evaluative perspectives from which interpretations are made. We say more about these supports to practical wisdom in the next section.

The discussion of practical wisdom is a reminder that the 'ethical expertise' of practitioners can be much broader than, and very different from, knowing about ethical theory. Practitioners who have been inducted into 'good habits' of improvement will be strongly disposed to find ways to steer health services towards greater effectiveness and safety whilst being mindful of the central importance of, and potential tensions with, other improvement purposes such as equity and person-centredness. They will have a grounded understanding of the context they are working in and be highly sensitive to the range of constituencies and voices that are invested in those contexts. They will have knowledge and experience about improvement approaches and, ideally, this will include a degree of scepticism, or at least caution, about whether they have a sound basis on which to act and an awareness that their actions carry practical and ethical risks. Where the official, informal and hidden curricula of education or workplace settings do not foster these kinds of habits, improvers should be asking if and how they might be reformed. To the extent these conditions are met there are reasons to be hopeful that the practical wisdom of improvement practitioners, enabled by currents embedded in the cultures and practices of the field, can provide a foundation for managing ethical issues in improvement.

But a focus on virtues and practical wisdom does not provide a straightforward answer, and cannot be the whole answer, to the challenges of improvement ethics. The previous paragraph presents a somewhat idealistic picture of professional practice. Financial, resource and time constraints can make it difficult or impossible to develop and maintain good habits and the educative and institutional structures needed to support them. But even setting such considerations aside, experienced and ethically conscientious professionals, even when working closely together facing the same scenarios, will sometimes be disposed to act in contrasting ways and there can be good reasons to debate the merits of, and the potentially relevant arguments that might be advanced to support, different inclinations and emphases. For example, healthcare improvement is characterized by a kind of 'two cultures' challenge – with strong scientistic currents sitting, sometimes relatively uncomfortably, alongside more humanistic ones.[25] These two emphases are liable to stress, respectively, different professional virtues – for example, the former may be more concerned with encouraging attitudes and habits of objectivity, meticulousness, precision and humility to research evidence, whereas the latter may emphasize flexibility, responsiveness, relational authenticity and humility to experience. Agreeing on the relevant set of virtues may itself present a series of controversies and uncertainties.

But, even where such tensions can be resolved, the diversity of improvers and improvement activities might mean that different virtues are more or less important depending on the individual in question, the role they are occupying at the time and the activities they are undertaking. Moreover, given that improvement requires consideration of multiple purposes, and can reflect the values and priorities of diverse groups and individuals, deep-seated ethical balancing acts and dilemmas will always lie just below the surface. This diversity includes a diversity of vantage points and a division of labour, as discussed in the previous chapter, between day-to-day practice on the ground and longer-term or more system-wide perspectives and responsibilities. Much more could be done to foster an awareness of this normative complexity, including sensitivity to the range of things that can be ethically salient, and to support practical judgement in healthcare improvement. In addition, there are questions to be asked about how well 'good habits' serve improvers when they are operating at different times, on different scales or in novel situations.

It is arguably good that a large proportion of the 'improvement workforce' consists of health professionals and that many of these are ethically literate, socialized into relevant professional virtues, deeply invested in their work and committed to offering good care. This professional expertise has important safeguarding potential, but we need to question its 'reach'. Relatively local and small-scale improvement activities might often be more or less 'covered' by the established virtues of clinical professionalism although, as we noted in the last chapter, even in small-scale improvement activities there are landscape and norm shaping purposes and effects that may need extra consideration. More ambitious, or larger-scale, improvement efforts by policymakers or other system leaders may call upon different kinds of thinking and capabilities – perhaps a different set of 'improvement virtues' – informed, for example, by debates in public health ethics and priority setting.

7.3 Encouraging listening and conversation

Fortunately, healthcare improvement does not rest wholly on the isolated judgement of individual practitioners. Rather it is a basic premise of improvement activity that it depends upon people working together, exchanging and comparing perspectives, and learning from one another. In this section we argue that these exchanges, though often taken for granted, are central to improvement ethics and a crucial mechanism through which different perspectives and normative complexity are recognized and managed in practice. In many cases, normative complexity is managed unselfconsciously but there are also cases where interactions can be specifically designed to acknowledge and tackle aspects of such complexity. This applies most obviously when weight is attached to consultation, or even 'co-production', with stakeholders including colleagues, patients and families.

This theme overlaps substantially with the two previous themes. Ethical accountability requires the sharing of accounts and perspectives. If it is to be a meaningful aspiration then, as we have argued, it has to be built upon a much broader culture of discussion and literacy about ethics. Indeed, arguably what matters more than one-off official 'stamps of approval' are the routine discussions that should take place amongst and between improvers and the people with whom, and for whom, they are working – discussions which could be seen as the continuous weaving of a web of 'mini-accountabilities'. Similarly, as we have highlighted, good habits and practical wisdom are fostered by various cultural and practical supports, amongst which are opportunities to talk with and learn from others.

Communication with, and not least listening to, other people is a fundamental component of 'data gathering' for improvement work. Being open to people's voices and values is not only an essential condition of being person-centred but also of any aspiration to consult with and respect stakeholders about the interpretation of, and perceived priorities with regard to, all dimensions of quality. These forms of engagement are now, for good reasons, seen as essential. In addition, talking and listening are fundamental components of improvement interventions – accounts of what is being suggested or done, and why, are an intrinsic part of the enactment of improvement. To talk about data collection is to rely on a research idiom but, obviously, not all the ways in which people learn about their environments need be thought about as research in any technical sense. Observing what happens in a particular health setting on a daily basis, having regular conversations with colleagues, managers, patients and people outside of work, generally having one's 'ear to the ground' and gaining experience of what it is like to work in a setting all provide rich insights and a 'feel' for institutions and systems which are highly valuable to improvers. Qualitative methods have a prominent place in improvement research and practice because they are one means of harnessing these insights, organizing and sharing them more widely, and complementing the often tidier-looking accounts offered by quantitative methods. Part of the business of qualitative methods is to take seriously diverse voices and perspectives and to embrace the relatively messy, anomalous and sometimes contradictory stories and snapshots that are elicited.[26] But it is equally important to recognize that more informal, everyday forms of listening and conversing also support healthcare improvement and good healthcare.

Here we say a bit more about what we mean by 'listening' and 'conversation', before reflecting on some of the broader ethical significance of listening and conversation, both as part of improvement interventions and in relation to the broader challenges of normative complexity and agenda setting.

Listening covers a spectrum of activities. It includes both informal attention to what colleagues, patients and other stakeholders are expressing, and formal information-gathering exercises that might be carried out by an institution or team. On the informal side, listening might take the form of managers and leaders attending to and taking seriously the concerns, ideas and complaints of their colleagues, including off-hand comments. Or it may involve staff who are in direct contact with patients – clinical professionals but also support staff such as porters, receptionists and volunteers – paying attention to the positive and negative feelings service users express (directly and indirectly) about health services and the care they receive. Informal views can be directly elicited or picked up on in the course of ordinary work. It is worth noting that both of these methods of data gathering carry epistemic risks: on the one hand, people may not always say what they really feel, if asked directly; on the other hand, staff may incorrectly interpret what colleagues and patients feel if they try to work it out from their actions, remarks, tone of voice, body language and so on. So both direct and indirect elicitation of views have the potential to mislead.

More formal methods of listening might involve more commonplace consultations and surveys, where typically the improvers who seek to know more about the perspectives, experience or knowledge of some population (usually staff, patients, families and carers, or/and the general public) determine the topic, questions, format and medium, and the responses of those surveyed are relatively constrained. But formal listening activities can also take more open-ended forms, which may be part of 'co-production' or 'experience-based co-design' activities that seek not just to ask stakeholders to provide information on pre-determined issues, but to partner with them at every stage including in thinking about what the most important topics and questions are, as well as how to answer them. More open-ended forms of listening present certain risks for institutions, because they have the potential to generate agendas and projects which are not aligned with existing plans, and they may challenge dominant framings and directives. If listening does generate such challenges, institutions may be put in a difficult position in deciding whether and how to act on them, especially if they are not aligned with financial and political incentives. If institutions have made grand claims about patient engagement and involvement, it may be particularly difficult to ignore or contradict the outcomes of such listening exercises without appearing to be hypocritical or engaged in vacuous and time-wasting activities.

The most open-ended listening exercises just discussed (as well as some of the more explicit informal listening exercises) may be more of a two-way street than the idea of 'listening' suggests, because meaningful engagement with colleagues, patients and other stakeholders can require conversation rather than just passive listening. Dialogical forms of engagement can also take a more informal or formal shape – compare a conversation that emerges naturally in the course of work with a discussion that has been planned and scheduled with the format or topic specified in advance. Conversations, including more facilitated or orchestrated ones, will always, however, be largely open ended. In general terms, a conversation is a reciprocal communicative exchange between two or more people, where perspectives, ideas and knowledge are shared. Conversations are characteristically not focused on some determinate end, such as coming to consensus or finding the truth on a matter – they do not necessitate any particular form of resolution. They are not decision-making procedures, though they may form a crucial part of decision-making.

In his illuminating account, Michael Oakeshott offers the following characterization of conversations:

> Conversation is not an enterprise designed to yield an extrinsic profit, a contest where a winner gets a prize, nor is it an activity of exegesis; it is an unrehearsed intellectual adventure. It is with conversation as with gambling, its significance lies neither in winning nor in losing, but in wagering. Properly speaking, it is impossible in the absence of a diversity of voices: in it different universes of discourse meet, acknowledge each other and enjoy an oblique relationship which neither requires nor forecasts their being assimilated to one another.[27]

This is arguably a description of a normative ideal, but we find it useful for highlighting several important features of conversations as a distinctive (and normative) communicative form. It would be too demanding to suggest that every instance of a conversation has all the features we highlight but we would suggest that good or paradigmatic conversations tend towards them. First, conversations are open-ended and their direction is not pre-determined. Second, they are not just debates or arguments, and do not have winners and losers. Third, they are not instrumentally directed towards particular ends, such as consensus or assimilation, nor do they require a definite resolution. Fourth, they meet some minimal conditions of respect – conversational partners acknowledge one another, recognizing the distinctive perspective and contributions that one another brings to the table, and regard one another with some minimal notion of relational equality. Thus understood, conversations have the capacity to contain and give voice to different and sometimes conflicting or contradictory perspectives without resolving tensions or coming to a judgement about them. While they may serve to change people's views and inform decision-making, they also have a vital non-instrumental value.

Both listening and dialogue can be thought about and justified in largely instrumental terms, and it may be tempting to do so in the context of such a practical activity as healthcare improvement. That is, listening and conversation are seen to be justified to the extent that they help to secure improvements, speed up the improvement process or generate improvements that are more sustainable or resilient to environmental shocks and changes. However, there are liable to be overlaps between instrumental and non-instrumental justifications of listening and conversation, insofar as these may only serve instrumental purposes well if they embody certain values, like respect and recognition.

One example of such an overlap is a justification for listening and conversation on the basis that they express respect for individuals. In much the same way as 'informed consent', and increasingly ideals and practices of clinician-patient collaboration, such as 'shared decision-making', are treated as core requirements in clinical ethics, it is reasonable to start from the presumption that something analogous should apply in healthcare improvement. This emphasis on consent for and engagement in improvement is reflected in the 'ethical requirements' listed by the Hastings Center project group discussed above (see Section 7.1). Identifying the appropriate kinds of mechanisms or informal processes for securing informed consent and collaboration might be problematic but the principle is relatively uncontroversial. It is arguably non-negotiable for moral actors to consider these principles if they are to treat any people that they are in a relationship with, and whose lives they are affecting or likely to affect, with respect. In a nutshell it means investing effort in finding out what matters to them and also ensuring they know about, understand and can help inform what is being proposed and how it will affect them. Listening and conversation are central to this. Such efforts may be justified in practice not just because they are ethically speaking the right thing to do, but also because they contribute to improvement activities that are responsive to the needs and preferences of service users and staff, not perceived as 'top-down' by those they affect, and informed by an understanding of what services are like 'on the ground'.

Openness to multiple voices and perspectives, whether based upon organic and informal presence, or more conscious and systematic qualitative research methods, is central to both effectiveness and ethics in improvement. It is relevant to the effectiveness of improvement efforts, as there is a danger that planned interventions will be misdirected or poorly designed if they miss significant features of a working context, including those that are difficult for people who are more removed from it to observe. Two-way dialogue is similarly vital – there is much greater likelihood that interventions will be initiated, sustained and whole-heartedly enacted by colleagues who have had a meaningful chance to discuss, question and help design and adapt them. Furthermore, the need to intervene may be missed altogether without conversations. For example, a crucial safety concern may be overlooked if systems are not able to pick up feelings of concern and intuitive worries that may fall below the radar of (and be in the wrong register for) formal reporting systems but surface as a result of informal talk and listening.[28]

Lying both behind and beyond these questions about effectiveness are questions about other ethical values. As discussed in Chapters 1 and 2 the question 'what works?' only fully makes sense when combined with the question 'what counts as working?' or slightly more expansively, 'what kinds and combinations of things are valuable in health and social care?' Much of this book has been taken up with highlighting normative complexity and thus showing why there is neither a simple nor a singular answer to these questions. We suggest that one foundational requirement for improvement ethics is for improvers to acknowledge and put themselves in a position to be open to this complexity. By listening to and conversing with other people and perspectives, improvers not only practise respect but also (a) expand their ethical awareness and (b) sensitize themselves to, confront and start to navigate the normative complexity of healthcare improvement. We discuss these in turn.

To accept the importance of listening is a stepping-stone to recognizing the broader ethical importance of perception, openness and sensitivity, including the ways these inform problem identification and definition.[29] Starting the analysis of ethical issues by focusing on proposed interventions is starting too late. Judgements about intervening, or not intervening, are grounded in judgements about what matters in specific times and places and from the vantage points of actors with different responsibilities, constraints and scope for action, as well as judgements about what counts as a relevant benchmark or ideal. When ascribing virtues and high levels of practical wisdom to people, part of what is being expressed is that they are ethically aware, responsive and discriminating in the way they experience and read their environment.

Things can go wrong when sensitivity to environments and climates is lacking from healthcare decision-making. For example, as is well known, serious harms can arise when healthcare institutions attach undue weight to particular targets. In the UK context this problem was given prominence by the report on major care scandals at Mid Staffordshire NHS Foundation Trust which set out the contribution of a target-driven climate.[30] This worry can be associated with some narrow managerial constructions of improvement, at least when they are not balanced with broader conceptions. But this is only an acute form of a more widespread potential risk of being captured by what we analysed in Part 2 as 'schematic' thinking, where what might be useful indications or operationalizations of quality and various quality dimensions are conflated with the whole picture. Once again there are valuable currents within the improvement field that can help reduce this risk and encourage a less constricted vision, and typically these have open-ended conversations and listening at the core.

One example, which aligns with placing some emphasis on multiple measures and soft intelligence already mentioned, is the development of an account of 'monitoring' alongside measurement in the patient safety field. Charles Vincent and colleagues developed a framework for maintaining the safety of healthcare settings expressly designed to move beyond over-reliance on specific tools (such as checklists) or techniques (such as 'safety huddles').[31] The framework is carefully elaborated and qualified but at its core it consists of five dimensions and associated questions:

1 *Past harms* – Has patient care been safe in the past?

2 *Reliability* – Are our clinical systems and processes reliable?

3 *Sensitivity to operations* – Is care safe today?

4 *Anticipation and preparedness* – Will care be safe in the future?

5 *Integration and learning* – Are we responding and improving?

The framework obviously requires translation into practice, but it is grounded in research on practice and has been studied in use, and the authors are clear that it needs to be adapted to context and to be co-constructed by engaged staff and patients. In a study of its implementation through a Canadian learning collaborative, practitioners were encouraged to engage in conversations about the framework and share it with colleagues without implementing any improvement interventions or producing deliverables.[32] Its value in broadening the gaze beyond targets alone was recognized, with one respondent (a senior leader) saying:

It's taught me that measuring refers to metrics and data, audits and count; whereas monitoring refers to the questioning, observing, listening, paying attention to people's perceptions. One of the big aha moments for me is in the past you set targets and so you're watching those targets and questioning when they're not being met and it really can lull you into a false sense of security when you're meeting those targets.[33]

This provides a plausible example of the kind of wide-ranging but still disciplined attention, fed by listening and conversation, that we are suggesting underpins ethical awareness.

Open-ended conversations and listening activities can help improvers to navigate the normative complexity of healthcare improvement. Being open to multiple sources of intelligence and voices from diverse standpoints should not be conflated with the project of finding consensus or constructing a shared position. Awareness is, in part, awareness of difference. It can make sense to forge common ground where possible, but consensus-building is only part of the value of extending awareness. There is much to be said for the value of conversations – both routine conversations and deliberately planned ones – even where these neither form part of the official institutional agenda or anyone's 'role description' nor come to any resolution or shared conclusion. Indeed it might be said that this lack of closure is precisely the special 'added value' of conversations.[34] Conversations – both between people working together in the same space and between people working at different institutional or system levels – allow for a range of positions to be 'contained together' without being collapsed into one another. Some people's voices and agendas will almost inevitably be relatively eclipsed by those of others in practice, but open discussion of different views will help improvers to recognize that conceptions and practices of improvement will not be equally satisfactory to everyone. There will also be ongoing tensions between actors with different priorities and/or who operate from different vantage points. All these actors may have a good claim to being ethically conscientious – indeed in many cases there may be no substantive ethical disagreements involved, just different agendas that do not neatly align. There is a close parallel here with what was said earlier about the commitment within (most versions of) qualitative research to represent and work with messy, anomalous and sometimes contradictory stories. Proceeding with an awareness of this messiness is substantially better than not doing so, not only because it better reflects genuine complexity but also because it can inflect how improvers behave and relate to others and how and when they may wisely recalibrate or even re-steer. Being aware of, and ideally attentive to, such divergence extends people's horizons and creates space for uncertainty. More broadly it helps foster moral imagination and empathy – essential components of any ethical toolkit.[35]

7.4 Turning to applied philosophy

Healthcare professionals and policymakers, including those with interests in improvement, sometimes turn to applied philosophers, most commonly those with an interest in healthcare ethics or bioethics, for guidance on ethical issues. Each of the three previous sections can be viewed as illustrating both that the field of healthcare improvement has existing practices to manage ethical issues and that these practices can be illuminated, and potentially strengthened by, engagement with philosophical perspectives. The challenge of accountability belongs to those who are practising improvement but the debates about determining appropriate expectations and applying models of accountability are informed by bioethicists as well as by senior improvement experts (as in the Hastings Center project). The exercise of good habits and institutional supports for practical wisdom must be 'built into' improvement practices and cultures but understanding the potential value and limitations of relying on ethical habits depends upon engagement with questions in philosophical ethics. Similarly, the kinds of attention and conversation we have highlighted need to be animated within, and to enlarge and enliven, improvement discourses but philosophical work is valuable in highlighting how and why they should be further fostered, and their centrality to ethics – in underpinning openness, empathy and moral imagination.

Philosophers, along to some extent with lawyers and religious studies experts, have assumed the position of ethics specialists or 'professionals'. In the case of philosophy, this makes sense because the very nature of ethics raises philosophical questions – such as questions about the scope and bases of ethics, the nature of ethical discernment and judgement including decision-making, and the possibility of offering ethical justifications in principle and in practice. It is typically philosophers who have developed and debated ethical theories or analyses which offer suggested answers to these kinds of questions and spent time debating the (in)adequacy of these theories. Obviously this does not mean that philosophers are 'better' at ethics in the sense that they are ethically better people, but it can mean that they are relatively comfortable with the multiple lenses and vocabularies of ethics and have significant literacy and some facility when it comes to articulating and unpacking the kinds of ethical dilemmas that can arise in health policy or clinical practice.

For that reason, applied philosophers have now become one part of the extended and diffuse community of expertise that populates health policy and services – working, for example, on professional codes of ethics, as members of commissions looking at challenging and/or novel topics and even, in some settings, as 'ethics consultants'.

Hopefully this chapter has made clear that there is more to ethics than philosophical ethics. Ethics cannot be 'contracted out' to philosophers or any other specialists. Philosophers can, however, be helpful partners or interlocuters and philosophical perspectives can also in some respects be incorporated within, and 'owned' by, healthcare actors including improvers. Indeed, this is arguably something that follows from any serious consideration of the nature of ethics: people are ethically responsible for what they do and, although they may benefit from advice, or reasonably defend themselves in situations where they are coerced or relatively powerless, they cannot transfer that ethical responsibility to someone else.

The rationale for the importance of dialogue, discussed in the last section, is, we suggest, relevant to exchanges and conversations between those active in healthcare improvement and those who are interested in applied philosophy (noting that these groups overlap). The same applies here as applies to a range of other groups – over time 'external' voices can, to varying degrees and in circumscribed respects, be integrated into a field. In the opening chapter we discussed the evolving contribution of sociology as an example. Another (of course only partial) analogue is the role of patients and carers in healthcare improvement. Both these examples indicate some of the tensions between the advantages of integration and those of critical distance. Philosophy, we are suggesting, can play a similar insider-outsider role.

We further elaborate the potential contribution of philosophy to healthcare improvement in Part 4 (and, of course, the whole book illustrates that contribution), but we can begin the elaboration here by briefly reviewing the roles of a philosophical partner or interlocuter in relation to improvement ethics. To do so we artificially separate out three broad functions that philosophical work can serve: (a) providing and strengthening resources, (b) offering and questioning 'big picture' accounts and (c) challenging and destabilizing prevailing discourses and practices. We should stress that this is an artificial separation, constructed from the perspective of a healthcare improvement interlocuter, and that there are no such clear boundaries within philosophy.

Philosophical work can help to furnish, maintain and hone the toolkit of improvement ethics. This applies, as we have illustrated, in relation to the themes discussed above. Concepts and theoretical frameworks – for example, related to accountability, consent, virtues, conversation and deliberation – can, to a significant extent, be 'borrowed from' the realm of applied philosophy and ethics where they are analysed, extensively debated and 'tested'. The same applies to many other value-laden ideas that have become prominent within improvement discourses, for example, concepts such as 'equality' or 'person'. Such concepts, as we have discussed, are not easy to 'pin down' (nor, we have suggested, should that always be our ambition). When improvers invoke them it is, for good reason, not always clear what is meant or implied. Philosophical work can play a key role here in encouraging an awareness of one's assumptions, opening up the range of ambiguity and contestation involved, asking for greater clarity about what is intended in particular cases and by noting the remaining indeterminacy (the notion here is analogous to a 'confidence interval' around probability estimates, for example, in studies of effectiveness: something important is added by making note of the presence and extent of indeterminacy). Here philosophy is constructed in a kind of service role. It provisions extra kit and helps to ensure that things in the ideas department go relatively smoothly or, where that is not possible, that potential clashes and crashes are anticipated.

A second way in which philosophy might support improvement ethics is arguably less modest and more 'visionary'. Applied philosophers can ask, and offer answers to, 'big picture' questions about concepts and values in ways that might usefully inform improvement ambitions and planning. For example, instead of asking improvement practitioners to examine the assumptions they happen to be making about their purposes, philosophers can start from posing very general questions such as questions about the purposes of medicine, health professions or health systems. Allied to this they can aim to develop general, useful and defensible accounts of concepts such as health and well-being. It should be obvious how this kind of work is relevant to improvement because it seems prima facie true to say that judgements about improving health systems, or healthcare practice, can to some extent be informed by thinking about, for example: (a) whether, or how far, underlying purposes are being adequately addressed and/or (b) whether central concepts built into practices are being interpreted and applied in ways that could be strengthened by recourse to more systematically elaborated accounts.

This may include thinking about how individual improvement projects support or detract from systemic values and aims.

This is not to assume that there would be agreement about possible 'big pictures' – likely there will not – nor that these can or should be easily and directly applied to resolving value uncertainties in healthcare improvement. But the articulation of over-arching systematic responses to these very general kinds of questions allows for the mapping of possible, plausible and competing visions of what healthcare improvement might look like. There should be no presumption of a 'top-down' translation or one-to-one mapping of philosophical accounts into improvement agendas. Moreover, improvement may, at least sometimes, legitimately start 'inside' healthcare with activities grounded in practical and ethical judgements about discernible, sometimes palpable, shortcomings or foreseeable gains. 'Big picture' accounts can at least provide useful heuristics, however, which can be profitably compared with particular versions of improvement in ways that stand to enhance the critical rigour underpinning both. (This is discussed further in Chapter 8.) Here philosophy is cast in a role as something of a 'thinking partner', enabling a particular form of dialogue and as a way of standing outside and stretching thinking, including practical wisdom, embedded in a professional or disciplinary field.

The third function of philosophical work that we have identified is roughly continuous with this 'thinking partner' account. That is, philosophers can act as critical friends – including sometimes as what might be thought of as 'constructively combative' friends. As mentioned in the opening chapter there are sceptical currents within healthcare improvement and one of the core functions of philosophy is to treat the business of scepticism very seriously. In relation to improvement ethics, this includes framing some very demanding, and potentially destabilizing, challenges and questions.

Scepticism here would include building on the kind of 'big picture' analyses just discussed to question whether prevailing approaches to improvement – in both conception and practice – fall short in fundamental ways, either being misdirected and partial or perhaps being positively harmful. The same sceptical lenses could be applied to both proposing and critically analysing radical revisionary agendas. At minimum this constructively combative approach would entail pressing home questions about what proportion of existing improvement activities are legitimate or ethically defensible. For instance, we earlier suggested that there is little reason, in general, to question the motivation of improvers. However, in practice there are cases where it seems that there are clear grounds to challenge this assumption. These grounds arise, for example, in contexts where engaging in improvement is a required part of training or otherwise imposed as a role expectation, rather than something that is responsive to identifiable deficits and needs. This worry might be generalized to include any set of circumstances where personal rewards – such as promotion or esteem – could result from engagement with improvement activities, or where scarce resources are deployed on improvement activities without careful consideration of the opportunity costs or the value and consequences of the activities themselves. There are many reasonable doubts about how far those practising improvement (a) know what they are doing and/or (b) are pursuing aims that would survive critical scrutiny. As we have stressed throughout our discussion, the existence of both explanatory and normative complexity mean that is difficult to know what combinations of intended and unintended effects will result from improvement activities and to assess the extent to which these should be variously regarded as desirable. In addition, as we have also noted, some relatively commonplace 'real-world' phenomena might reasonably serve to reinforce rather than damp down scepticism about improvement activities. These include, for example, harnessing improvement discourses to serve the (typically narrower) managerial agendas of institutions, or the tendency, despite good efforts, for some perspectives and voices to be relatively marginalized in the design of planned interventions.

Although it is tempting to present these three stories about the possible benefits of engagement with applied philosophy as on a spectrum from relatively 'insider' to 'outsider' accounts, the truth is that each can be constructed with more of an emphasis on incorporation or critique. In each case, there are strong resonances with perspectives and concerns already being articulated within healthcare improvement. This certainly includes heavily sceptical and critical voices from those practically invested in the field.[36] In this regard asking hard, philosophically inspired, questions about how to strengthen improvement and improvement ethics can be understood as a helpful support and stimulus, as having some liberatory potential and as a call for greater care, rigour and creativity.

A sign of a robust, mature professional domain is that it can find space for, and indeed welcome and actively seek, input from, partnership with and challenge from others. In the case of improvement ethics we suggest that these exchanges are invaluable for cultivating the kinds of ethical literacy and dialogue that the Hastings Center report envisages growing as part of a climate that enables appropriate forms of accountability. We have sought to stress that there are already resources and practices in healthcare improvement that help to underpin the ethical bases and defensibility of the field. At the same time the ethical significance of these resources is not widely recognized and there is much to be gained both by highlighting this significance and by more self-consciously examining, enriching and challenging these 'built-in' resources. We are, of course, not envisaging some one-off transformation and certainly not downloading an ethics upgrade from the philosophy store. Nor are we imagining that everyone engaged in improvement work should constantly be having all the conversations we have discussed. In this case, as elsewhere, there must be some division of labour. Mapping a division of labour for improvement ethics would be daunting but we can offer a simple dichotomy as a starting point: on-the-ground improvement practitioners should be increasingly supported and prepared to offer an ethically reflective account of the complications that arise from their endeavours. At the same time, within policy debate and in professional education there should be space for 'root-and-branch' questioning of healthcare improvement agendas and practices, including potential downfalls, associated harms and ethical dilemmas. Of course, there should be cross-fertilization between these two kinds of discussion, and many improvers will be well-placed to participate in and contribute to both.

In this concluding section we have presented engagement with philosophy and ethics as one means of extending and strengthening debate and the scope of accountability in healthcare improvement. But, more fundamentally, across the chapter, we have argued that accountability in a richly meaningful sense requires a routinely dialogical and critically self-reflexive improvement community. Healthcare improvement is grounded in, and contributes to, a sceptical and questioning approach to health systems and practices. Improvers are continuously asking whether systems and practices are fit for purpose and how they might be made better. This involves helping to articulate the rationale of services and questioning whether, and the extent to which, existing provision can be defended. This critical distance from the system is invaluable but it needs extending into a second-order form of criticality. Being oriented towards and practising improvement is not sufficient. Rather the same critical ethical scrutiny needs to be applied to the construction and enactment of healthcare improvement itself. As set out in the previous chapter, improvers, consciously or not, effectively make up a body of healthcare legislators. This entails that the scope of their critical reflection and ethical debate needs to extend widely and encompass the strengths and weaknesses of competing framings of the 'what' and 'how' of improvement and not just the merits and shortcomings of health services.

PART FOUR

RETHINKING IMPROVEMENT

8 RADICAL IMPROVEMENT

Healthcare improvement is, by definition, about changing things. Sometimes the improvements that matter will require major rethinking of the way healthcare is organized and practised. This possibility – which forms the focus of this chapter – corresponds with the idea of revisionary improvement perspectives introduced in Chapter 1. Although we have resisted drawing a firm line between delivery and revisionary perspectives, the distinction points to the idea that as well as finding ways to refine and better execute existing healthcare processes and practices, improvement might include changing the way the rationale of healthcare is conceived, including perhaps even its core purposes and norms.

In the previous two chapters, and to some extent throughout the book so far, we have stayed relatively close to a delivery perspective. This is because we often have in mind healthcare improvement as a professional domain and a delivery perspective is arguably closer to the mainstream of the field. Improvement and implementation sciences emphasize feasible and measurable changes including better delivery of established or emerging evidence about 'what works' and what stands a chance of being replicable in other settings. These emphases tend to limit how open-ended and ambitious improvement agendas can be. But, as we have noted before, even mainstream versions of improvement contain revisionary elements. For example, calls for more person-centred and equal ways of relating, although now relatively standard, often embody a demand that healthcare norms need further revision. Other currents within the improvement field also signal far-reaching or ambitious agendas, including the concern with 'scaling up' improvements and thus with change at scale – sometimes described in terms of system 'transformation' or rolling out 'innovations'. This suggests we might think of ambition in terms of breadth and/or depth, that is for widespread (albeit sometimes minor) change and/or for a change to underlying assumptions and norms.[1] In this chapter we are, for the most part, interested in 'depth' and the idea of 'radical improvement' as signalling changes to healthcare roots as well as branches, but we will also keep breadth in mind and say a little more about it in the concluding section of the chapter. Before that we will explore 'roots' – or underlying assumptions – in two ways. In the next section we discuss some examples of work in philosophy of health that focus on potential 'first principles' for rethinking healthcare. Following that we discuss two specific real-world examples of revisionary framings of good healthcare: that healthcare should be 'sustainable' and 'anti-racist'.

8.1 What is healthcare for?

One starting point for more radical ways of constructing improvement is to look at critical or novel accounts of the aims or potential contributions of healthcare. If someone arrives at the conclusion that healthcare should be serving ends 'abc' but in practice it serves ends 'xyz' then they may judge that a fundamental reorientation is called for. This kind of judgement is familiar in specific practical contexts, when a patient feels that what a service offers them is quite different from what they consider they need, and in more sweeping complaints, for example, that institutions provide a 'sickness service' rather than a 'health service'. Several more conceptually and theoretically systematic positions have also been proposed that set out a possible basis for healthcare reorientation. This is one of the ways that academic philosophers have contributed to discussions about healthcare. There is an influential approach to applied philosophy – that also features in other areas such as philosophy of education – that springs from asking abstract and fundamental questions about the nature of the object of investigation. These questions could include, for example: 'What is health?' 'What is the purpose of healthcare?' 'What goods should healthcare serve?' Within this approach such questions are asked primarily as questions about concepts and ethics – questions about the meaning of health-related concepts and the potential role of healthcare in contributing to individual and collective well-being – rather than as empirical questions about how, as a matter of fact, words are used in a particular context or what, in practice, gets done. The results of these theoretical investigations may differ quite starkly from the practical realities of how institutions function and how their function is understood by most people. This 'gap' helps to explain the critical potential of asking the fundamental questions: they can help people to think about how things might be different from and perhaps better than the status quo.

A brief example from philosophy of education can illustrate the point. A philosophical analysis of the nature and aims of education might conclude that education is, in some significant measure, about developing and supporting the autonomy of learners – that is, providing people with the knowledge, character qualities and learning pathways to help enable them to chart their own way through life. Assuming something like this is part of someone's considered conclusion, this would provide a basis for them to critique existing educational provision, highlighting concerns, for example, about pedagogical approaches that are in some ways 'knowledge rich' (in that they include a lot of 'subject content') but which rely on relatively narrow conceptions of what counts as knowledge and pay insufficient attention to the broader factors that support the development of autonomy. On this account such approaches might not only fall short of an ideal of education but even do harm. Working from 'first principles' in this way might not only motivate critique but also help enable theorists and practitioners to sketch out some characteristics of an alternative and better model. Before considering how this kind of reasoning about fundamentals or 'first principles' can be, and has been, applied to healthcare we should note that philosophical analysis does not have to start from outside practice. Strongly overlapping insights can arise from work in philosophy and other critical disciplines that starts closer to practice and identifies existing concerns, perspectives and values that some people acknowledge as important but that are generally neglected.

A relatively common factor in critical analyses of healthcare within philosophy (and other vantage points) is a worry about the limiting or 'distorting' influence of the powerful biomedical model on the constitution of healthcare. As discussed in Part 2, a biomedical vision of healthcare might conceive of its purpose in terms of the identification and treatment of pathology, and the restoration of normal physical and psychological function: health is understood as the absence of disease or physiological abnormality. The worry expressed by critical philosophical analyses can start from the idea that the biomedical model captures just some of what matters for healthcare and risks conflating means and ends because it focuses on processes such as combatting disease or treating pathology rather than asking what goods motivate these processes. The distorting influence of biomedical model thinking is illuminated by contrast with philosophically elaborated and defended alternatives. For example, some philosophers have offered positive accounts of the nature and value of health, over and above the absence of disease, which suggest broader aims for healthcare than wholly biomedical ones. Overlapping with these are accounts which emphasize the intersections between healthcare and public health, the role of health in contributing to social opportunities and fairness, the place of 'care' in healthcare, and some of the relational, meaning-giving and experiential goods that healthcare serves. Our concern here is neither to critically evaluate, nor add to, these accounts; rather, we are interested in highlighting their potential for challenging prevailing conceptions of healthcare and informing revisionary perspectives. We start by giving a slightly fuller indication of some examples. To clarify we are not offering these as rival candidates for a singular correct account of the nature of healthcare; rather we suggest that, taken together, they illuminate key considerations and contribute to an understanding of health and healthcare as a contested domain.

Some philosophers have proposed accounts of health as a positive good in contrast to the absence of biomedically defined disease or disability, or to the personal experience of illness. For example, David Seedhouse characterizes health as the 'foundations for achievement': someone is healthy to the extent that they are in conditions that enable them to realize their 'biological and chosen potentials'.[2] Lennart Nordenfelt argues for a broadly similar definition of health, as 'the ability, in standard circumstances, to realize [one's] vital goals, i.e., the set of goals which are necessary and together sufficient for [one's] minimal happiness'.[3] Nordenfelt's definition suggests a threshold for what qualifies as being healthy and thus for the range of relevant conditions, whereas Seedhouse leaves the notion of health and the idea of foundations as highly elastic, but both accounts present health as something which includes but transcends biomedically defined functioning.

Such accounts of health have important practical and normative implications. Any picture of satisfactory healthcare which takes them seriously is likely to place an emphasis on 'health promotion', interpreted as something more than the prevention of disease. For example, responses from health professionals to people living in poverty conditions (as in the case study reviewed in Chapter 2) can be seen not simply as allied to treatment or prevention of disease but as another aspect of the enterprise of promoting people's health by enabling them to live their lives and pursue non-health-related aims and interests. Likewise, the role of 'health visitors' will not be understood as valuable for health only because it helps underpin physiological development and biological functioning but also because it helps enable parents to navigate social challenges and manage day to day.[4] These philosophical accounts of 'positive health' are clearly value-laden because they depend on conceptions of what constitutes human achievement and/or happiness. These normative pictures can be contrasted with the idea – supported by some – that it is possible to give a largely value-neutral, or 'non-normative', definition of health in biomedical terms and thus, perhaps, for the core purposes of health professionals to be scientifically specified. This view is represented, most famously, in Christopher Boorse's 'biostatistical conception' of health which defines health in terms of biology and 'statistical normality', but also attracts contemporary advocates.[5]

The normative nature of the value-laden 'extra-biomedical' accounts we have summarized can therefore be seen at two levels. First, if the way actors frame healthcare is explicitly based on interpretations of human purposes and values, then there can be no question but that the 'core business' of health-related work is normatively constructed. Second, the specific content of a philosophical account of health (e.g. the construction of 'achievement' or 'happiness' or other 'endpoints', and the accompanying account of the role of health in a good society) will have differing implications for the exact ways in which professionals, policymakers and citizens conceive and evaluate healthcare and health policy.

More recently philosophers have proposed accounts of health and healthcare that stress the centrality of public health perspectives to all aspects of health policy including the organization and conduct of healthcare. For example, Sridhar Venkatapuram argues that an understanding of the nature of health, and the widely endorsed notion of a 'right to health', in the terms he sets out and defends, entail radical shifts for health policy.[6] Venkatapuram's account of health critically responds to and seeks to offer greater specification and consistency to the animating idea behind Nordenfelt's definition. Drawing on the influential 'capabilities approach' he defines health in terms of the 'capability to be healthy' which depends on having the kind of range of real opportunities needed to achieve well-being.[7] He argues that ensuring everyone has such opportunities is ethically warranted both to reflect and support human dignity and to give people the chance to build a life that is valuable to them. Venkatapuram's approach can highlight the very substantial within-country and global disparities in circumstances and opportunities and illuminate the challenges of realizing social justice in relation to health. Thinking about 'care for health' in this frame exposes the risk that even ambitions for universal access to healthcare services may not add up to much if many people's life settings make it systematically less likely that they can access such services and much more likely that they need them.

Sean Valles' 'Philosophy of Population Health' also stresses public health perspectives, including the social determinants of health inequalities but additionally argues that health is inherently social.[8] That is, not only do the causes and effect of health experiences need to be understood, investigated and addressed in social terms, but individual and community health should be understood as inherently co-constitutive. In Valles' terms, health is 'metaphysically social' – social in nature or in its very being. Valles uses this social conception of health to argue that much contemporary healthcare has been sent in a wrong, and sometimes, harmful direction by the influence of a biomedical conception of health which has led, for example, to excessive use of technologies and clinical interventions that either do not collectively improve population health or even risk worsening it.

There are echoes in the tone of Valles' philosophical critique of prevailing health services of the constructively combative way Seedhouse offered his 'foundations of achievement' account of health as 'a gauntlet' to throw 'at the feet of those responsible for the organization and delivery of health care'.[9] Someone persuaded by one or more of these philosophical analyses of the nature of health and role of healthcare may well resolve that radical change is required to improve healthcare. Before turning to that idea, we briefly mention another important example of a fundamental philosophically based challenge – one that also draws a contrast with dominant biomedical thinking, but with a different emphasis.

Work drawing on phenomenology directs our attention to health as it is experienced, so-to-speak, 'from the inside'. From this perspective one of the key shortcomings of thinking about ill-health purely biomedically is that this misses the lived experience of sickness, illness and disability. Havi Carel has elucidated a rich account of the importance of understanding and responding to illness in these terms.[10] To experience illness (understood as something more than a short-term bout of sickness) involves managing different relationships with other people, with time and space, with one's own past and future, as well as with one's body. It requires people to work on many aspects of their identity and to confront mortality. In many ways this is the substance of illness, but it is a substance that is not touched by biomedical science. Responding to it adequately only starts when we engage with first-person perspectives and the reality of subjective experience. In some respects, it looks as if there is a contrast between Valles' emphasis on the social dimension and Carel's emphasis on the personal and the first-person dimension. But it is arguably better to see them as offering contrasting emphases on the social realm. Personal experiences are socially shaped, and both contend that meaningful responses to illness need to be interpersonal and social. Phenomenological approaches emphasize the value of engaging with people's narratives, bearing witness to their suffering and working with them to help reshape their biographies and sense of who they are.

We want to reiterate the spirit in which we are presenting these very brief summaries of philosophical work. We are definitely not suggesting that any of them should be accepted and adopted uncritically. In a sense, philosophical work is developed to be critically taken apart. As already noted, these accounts are often, in part, formulated in opposition to one another and, even when not, they are typically accompanied by a critical literature which, amongst other things, suggests ways in which the premises, lines of reasoning and conclusions of other accounts are inadequate or flawed. What we are highlighting is that it is possible and can be productive to ask, in a systematic and sustained way, about the fundamental nature of health and the possible purposes of healthcare. If, after applying due criticality, it is possible to establish that an account (or some combination of accounts) is credible and reasonably robust, this may help illuminate the grounds and directions of necessary healthcare change.

It is not necessary to imagine that such a foundational philosophical account could provide a clear 'blueprint' for the development of a whole healthcare system. There will be an indefinite number of ways – including better and worse ones – of realizing theoretical framings of health and the purposes of healthcare in practice. But such accounts might nonetheless be valuable lenses that can help people see and 're-see' the strengths and weaknesses of health-related practices and policies. We reiterate that similar philosophical insights can arise and be developed in more 'bottom up', and sometimes more ad hoc, ways and can be found and integrated within work in other disciplines (we say more about this in Chapter 9). Many of the concerns summarized above have parallels in routine and lively debates *within* healthcare. But it is worth investigating the thought that if some of the central assumptions, concepts and constructions of purpose that shape healthcare *are* mistaken then improvement may require pervasive changes to working models – to the 'logic' of practices rather than simply to the way practices are delivered.

In the following sections we look more closely at some examples of ways in which healthcare might be reoriented – by making commitments to sustainability and anti-racism more central. But first, to set the scene, we quickly sketch out the potential radicalism of substantially reframing healthcare and note some of the possible objections to doing so, by drawing on themes we have discussed in earlier chapters. We begin with the suggestion that healthcare should be oriented towards, or much more oriented towards, population health rather than largely towards successful delivery of health service interventions and treatments. This could be interpreted in several ways but let us suppose that it includes healthcare professionals constructing their roles in ways that makes them more sensitive and responsive to health inequalities and social determinants of health such as poverty. The suggestion might also justify a shift in focus from short-term clinical outcomes towards longer-term health and well-being. These imagined changes would presumably entail those responsible for running health services looking at the way those services' economic, social and cultural resources and influence can be used to help tackle health inequalities.[11] In many respects and in significant measure this seems uncontentious. Given the working assumptions that health services exist to give people a greater chance of being well rather than unwell, and that everyone should be equally entitled to this chance (not uncontentious but widely accepted) then increasing health service orientation towards population health in these ways seems something close to a mere step in logic.

This way of 'resetting healthcare', we suggest, could have radical implications not only for the aims of healthcare improvement but also for its approaches and methods. It seems clear that the aims of healthcare improvement would have to expand. Existing health services that might hitherto have been seen as doing an adequate or good job will be judged to be falling short in some way – here, for example, by insufficiently addressing health inequalities. But it also seems to follow that the character of improvement work might need to change substantively, shifting its centre of gravity from looking to understand, refine and spread 'successful' healthcare practices to routinely looking at such practices with a critical eye, and looking outside healthcare and the scope of health professionals' work to imagine other policies and practices that might better tackle poverty and health inequality. In this scenario the SDOH screening case study discussed in Chapter 2 would be a relatively minor example of mainstream work rather than an added extra, and the overall exercise would be one of large-scale re-education and structural transformation. Changing the sense of direction seems bound to require changes to approaches and methods. First, it involves a shift in perception, with different features of the healthcare landscape becoming salient – as previously unproblematic elements become problematic. Second it makes it likely that improvers will have to reconceive starting points and modes of action. In the 'population well-being-oriented' case imagined here, for example, a good deal of the focus of improvement work would have to be turned beyond clinic walls and to effective means of building and strengthening social policies and partnerships that tackle the determinants of health.

However, it is not difficult to see potential hazards with shifting the improvement agenda in this way. Indeed, it is important to raise questions about how far such a 'resetting' makes sense and is defensible. Most obviously there is a risk of breaking things under the guise of fixing things. In efforts to promote alternative, more radical, ideas there may be a tendency to downplay or lose sight of the value of whatever is thereby being subverted. In other words, there is a danger of 'throwing the baby out with the bathwater'. In such contexts, the monitoring of 'unintended effects', which is helpfully advocated in several currents of improvement thinking, requires more wide-ranging attention and work. By way of analogy, let's imagine someone was to analyse the activities of a community bookshop and conclude that the bookshop is valuable because it provides the community with education, entertainment and an accessible and friendly culturally enriching meeting place. We might also suppose that the bookshop owner is keen to serve the community in an inclusive way and stocks a broad range of books for diverse audiences including large print and audiobooks. If a would-be improver came along and suggested that for the bookshop to properly serve its apparent mission it needed to organize more social events, offer more and more basic literacy education and use a large proportion of the space it occupies to offer an extensive programme of film viewing, dance and music, what would we think? It is quite possible that we could believe that this new agenda was a persuasive and important one but, at the same time, we worry that many of the things the bookshop did well would be damaged or completely lost in the process. We might even think that the improvement proposal involved it ceasing to be a bookshop altogether.

The bookshop analogy suggests that, even if healthcare services do and should, in some measure, adopt some public health priorities, there might be limits to how far this makes sense and can be defended. Taking the analogy to heart might lead someone to think that there are a distinct set of goods that healthcare services provide – perhaps something like responding to the needs of the acutely sick and those with long-term illness by providing them with treatments and care – and that the reliable provision of these goods need to be protected from 'improvements' directed at other things, even if these are construed as somehow also meeting the same ends. This is not, at base, a worry specific to public health priorities. The same concern could arise, for example, with a 'radical improvement' programme based upon strengthening aspects of person-centred care. An improver might be sufficiently persuaded by the plausibility of placing illness (understood phenomenologically) rather than disease (understood biomedically) centre stage that they advocate for substantially greater focus on more meaningful healthcare relationships, closer attention to illness narratives and far greater support for managing 'biographical disruption'.[12] Others might reasonably believe that these newly emphasized imperatives are all worthwhile but also have a legitimate concern about whether a programme designed to shift healthcare in this direction might significantly undermine the provision of other existing goods.

One way that these worries about 'radical improvement' might be articulated is by suggesting that strong boundaries should be drawn between healthcare and other more broadly conceived health-related activities and goods. The boundaries would help signal the distinctiveness of healthcare and, at a practical level might, for example, help prevent doctors and other health professionals from having 'external' agendas and perspectives foisted upon them to the detriment of their 'core job'. For reasons we will soon clarify, we want to resist the notion that such definite boundaries can be drawn or are necessarily helpful. The example of person-centred care suggests another way of constructing the tensions under consideration here. As we argued in Part 2, if the notion of 'quality' or 'good healthcare' is plural and contested then it follows that attempts to provide good healthcare, or to improve healthcare, will routinely involve becoming aware of and managing tensions and trade-offs between multiple aspects of (and vantage points on) good-quality healthcare. There is always a risk of would-be improvers over-emphasizing something they judge to be valuable. A service that was configured just to concentrate on listening to and 'hearing' the experience of ill people (and/or to 'simply' be responsive to their preferences, to take another aspect of person-centred care) might be a very bad service in other key respects. But, we suggest, no mainstream health policymaker or manager faced with these tensions would argue that the best way of handling them would be to situate key aspects of person-centredness beyond the boundaries of healthcare or to see them as falling wholly outside 'core activities' and as mere 'nice to haves'. This example also highlights that what counts as inherent to a particular service evolves over time and, as discussed in the opening chapters, is shaped by changing social norms and expectations, including changing (professional and community) knowledge about and conceptions of health and suffering.

8.2 Sustainability and evolving improvement priorities

In this and the following section we consider two examples of potential revisionary agendas for healthcare improvement: (environmental) sustainability and anti-racism. These represent areas in which some, and arguably most, healthcare services might be judged to be falling short or failing, and therefore areas for improvement. This claim can be made with plausibility today but might have gone largely unrecognized thirty years ago when the field of healthcare improvement was only beginning to coalesce. The questions the sustainability and anti-racism agendas raise overlap with those discussed in Section 8.1 in relation to the foundations of improvement thinking and the social ends impacted by health-related work. At the same time, they both have some clear continuities with conventionally recognized 'dimensions' of healthcare quality, including efficiency and equity. How might the increasing incorporation of such agendas change the field? In what follows we argue that these concerns need to be included within improvement research and practice but have substantial potential to disrupt and help reorient improvement discussions and cannot be 'added on' in a simple way. This latter is because neither of these concerns – sustainability or anti-racism – has a single determinate meaning and taking them seriously involves managing tensions in both interpreting their implications and integrating them with other considerations.

The discussion in Section 8.1, we suggest, indicates why it is problematic to simply resist these frame-enlarging agendas. Taking the idea of sustainability to start with, it is certainly possible to argue that sustainability might not be considered a core purpose of healthcare in the same way that some accepted 'quality concepts', like effectiveness and safety, might be. But, first, that is clearly not the same as arguing that sustainability is not a relevant consideration for evaluating healthcare and second, there seems to be no good reason to imagine that improvement activities should only be aimed at core purposes. Any resistance here risks committing the basic practical and ethical mistake of imagining that healthcare should be judged only in terms of the good that it is intended to do rather than also in relation to the harms or wrongs that it might directly or indirectly bring about.

The sense in which 'sustainability' has, up until recently, been most often discussed in the quality improvement literature refers to the longevity of improvement benefits. It may be that some improvement efforts bring about desired benefits in terms of better healthcare in the short term, but what can be done to increase the chance that these benefits persist when the visible improvement efforts are over or, rather perhaps, fade into the background? *The Institute for Healthcare Improvement* has developed a worksheet to support this kind of sustainability, and academic work has been done which helps theorize its bases and inform practice.[13] This longevity-of-benefit sense of sustainability links directly into a broader, more umbrella, sense where sustainability refers to capacity to continue some activity and produce some good. Appeals within institutional life to consider long-term financial sustainability are familiar examples of this usage. Such appeals require health policy actors to attend to cost-effectiveness over an extended period, including, for example, to be cautious about introducing novel, highly expensive technologies which may have indeterminate or small population benefits as well as opportunity costs elsewhere. There are ways in which this idea of long-term sustainability is simply continuous with mainstream notions in healthcare improvement. An activity designed to underpin good-quality healthcare may not be effective if it only has short-term effects, and such time-limited effects can be seen as wasteful of resources and thus inefficient. Embracing sustainability might thus be viewed as adopting slightly wider and longer-term views on what counts as success, adjusting the parameters to consider interests beyond those of current patients and other immediate beneficiaries.

The language of sustainability is arguably now used most often, and in a wide range of policy contexts, to refer to environmental sustainability. This too can be related to the very general umbrella notion where sustainability means something like not pursuing immediate ends in ways that fail to address, or positively undermine, the ability to continue to meet the same ends over time. It is possible to draw a continuous line between the quite circumscribed idea of sustaining improvement effects and the more global concerns of environmental sustainability although the emphases as we move along the line shift substantially. A team of health professionals who want to protect the quality of the service they offer will need to look weeks, months and sometimes years ahead to check whether there are reliable sources of medicines, equipment, trained staff and so on, and to be mindful about potential deterioration of service infrastructures. Any service, however modest and targeted it is, depends upon an extensive network of technical, cultural, social and economic activities, resources and systems. Environmental sustainability is concerned with what is needed to maintain and preserve the background supporting conditions, resources and systems, including at a global level and often with an emphasis on diminishing natural resources and a planetary ecosystem that is under threat from factors such as pollution and climate change. In one sense, then, these two interpretations of sustainability connect – although they refer to different timeframes and scales of resources and systems. However, the move towards environmental sustainability seems, roughly speaking, to involve shifting from matters that seem largely 'internal' to planning health services to ones that seem largely 'external' – at least in the short-to-medium term. This distinction is sometimes reflected in economic discourse using the language of 'externalities' – those costs (and benefits) of activity that are not typically included within models of institutional effectiveness and efficiency which consider only circumscribed and 'institutionally located' costs and benefits.

Environmental sustainability, and especially the threat of climate change, is now relatively high on health policy agendas and, albeit to a lesser extent, gaining prominence within health service quality improvement. A key theme of discussion is the substantial public health damage threatened by, and in some places already in train from, climate change. An emphasis on the determinants of health (and disease and death) seems to place this agenda beyond the scope of healthcare as conventionally understood, but there are some respects in which this is not the case. First, given these substantial health risks and costs, doctors and other health professionals have a role, and arguably a duty, to lobby for national and international cross-government and inter-governmental strategies to combat climate change.[14] Dominant amongst these are strategies designed to reduce carbon emissions into the atmosphere. Second, because health professionals are relatively influential and trusted members of society, they have a role in helping to communicate about the relevant risks and mitigations to patients and the public. Third, as workers within a sector that consumes considerable resources and contributes to environmental damage, including through carbon emissions, they can strive – alongside health policymakers, managers and other staff – to directly reduce this negative impact and thereby help address the environmental determinants of ill-health.

Relatively high-profile examples of policy actions in this area include the American Medical Association (AMA) declaring climate change a public health crisis in 2022. A Board spokesperson was quoted as saying:

> The scientific evidence is clear, our patients are already facing adverse health effects associated with climate change, from heat-related injuries, vector-borne diseases and air pollution from wildfires, to worsening seasonal allergies and storm-related illness and injuries. Like the COVID-19 pandemic, the climate crisis will disproportionately impact the health of historically marginalized communities.[15]

The AMA called for those working in medicine and the healthcare sector to decarbonize, including by reducing consumption of fossil fuels and looking for alternatives to the petroleum-derived plastics used in medical devices and products. In a related press release they noted that 'the U.S. health care sector is responsible for an estimated 8.5 percent of national carbon emissions and 25 percent of global health sector emissions'.[16]

Comparable stances have been taken in other countries. In the UK, for example, the Royal College of Physicians (RCP) has been advocating for action on climate health for many years and in 2023 added sustainability and climate change to its list of core policy and campaign priorities.[17]

The RCP's recommendations are largely directed at governmental cross-sectoral strategy and action on climate change and public health (ranging from reducing fossil fuels, tackling air pollution, shifts from private car use to walking, cycling and public transport, and promotion of green spaces) but also include recommendations focused on the UK NHS in particular, to help meet a target of it becoming net zero in emissions by 2040. Accounts of the contribution that healthcare makes to environmental and public health harms – for example that the NHS is responsible for 4 per cent of total UK emissions – show the clear relevance of environmental sustainability to healthcare quality improvement.

The corollary of the idea that healthcare organizations are 'anchor institutions' – institutions in a position to deploy social, political and economic influence to help address public health needs including health inequalities in communities and regions – is that they can be responsible for substantial damage.[18] It is a central feature of both clinical healthcare and improvement approaches to pay attention to 'side effects' and 'costs'. All action is complex; as well as hopefully bringing about intended effects, actions are inevitably also bound up in other causal chains that produce unintended or unforeseen effects. The implications of healthcare for the environment are very substantial, and historically often unrecognized or ignored, side effects or costs.

This takes us to the predominant way in which environmental sustainability has been adopted in the field of healthcare improvement. Those improvers who have advocated for its inclusion have typically presented damage to the environment as an extra cost that should be taken into account when considering the costs and benefits of changing healthcare. For example, an Institute of Healthcare Improvement blog which recommends integrating environmental sustainability into healthcare quality and safety work begins by summarizing how climate change can adversely affect the (conventional six) aims of quality improvement and then proposes, for example, that improvers should prioritize improvement or implementation projects that both advance healthcare quality *and* result in lower carbon emissions.[19] Here carbon emissions are treated like a form of waste – 'active waste' – and keeping sustainability in mind can lead to efficiency savings, where the same or more health benefit could be created with less cost or damage. This parallel with reducing waste is also prominent in an early proposal for making sustainability a 'pillar' of improvement, published as an editorial in *BMJ Quality & Safety*, which argues that the NHS carbon reduction measures are supporting efficiencies and have potential to produce large financial savings across all health systems.[20]

The Centre for Sustainable Healthcare in the UK has developed an approach to sustainable healthcare quality improvement that draws on various roots and combines them into a systematic account of 're-valuing' what counts as good quality healthcare. The Centre's broad principles of sustainable healthcare echo those signalled in other policy papers – including more concentration on prevention, the empowerment and mobilization of patients including through self-care, 'lean' clinical pathways, and finding and implementing low carbon alternatives to existing provision. The value of healthcare is still approached as a function of 'benefits' over 'costs' but the Centre adopts a 'triple bottom line' approach that explicitly redefines (sustainable) value as the benefit of outcomes for patients and populations set against the sum total of environmental, social and financial impacts.[21]

Reframing the valuation of healthcare, and thus what counts an improvement, has significant ethical and practical effects that the Centre recognizes and advances. The approach encourages people to take an expansive and inclusive way of thinking about improvement, including seeing healthcare aims as closely interwoven into other social aims that cannot be separated out without illogical consequences. In addition, it re-energizes improvement motivations sparked by sustainability as a new quality concern, encourages attention to 'future-proofing' (sustainability in the sense initially discussed above), increases the salience of opportunities to reduce harmful environmental and social impacts, and stimulates the monitoring and measurement of sustainability benefits which can be communicated widely to highlight both their importance and what is possible. This approach has been extensively shared and adopted in a range of sites. An illustrative case study shows, for example, how changing the model of care in a cardiac intensive care unit by preparing patients for earlier discharge into community and self-care had benefits for both patients and staff and, at the same time, saved over 1 million pounds sterling and almost 50 tonnes of carbon emissions over a two-year period.[22]

It would be difficult to argue against the broad logic illustrated in this and similar case studies. If improvers use the lens and motivation offered by a sustainability agenda to look for ways to reduce interventions or re-model services so that the same (or better) 'goods' can be achieved using fewer resources, this can only be seen as a spur to quality improvement.

In these instances, sustainability serves not only as a way of increasing efficiency and safety (by replacing or reducing 'unproductive' or positively harmful healthcare activities) but also of broadening improvers' gaze such that they become more mindful of the broader social and economic impacts of health services, including on population and planetary health. These cases broadly correspond with the 'both and' features of examples used in the IHI blog mentioned above.[23] Put another way they relate to instances where sustainability is 'added in' to improvers' general way of conceiving of and pursuing healthcare quality. But this construction faces important conceptual, ethical and empirical challenges. For example, there are plausible readings of the idea and principles of sustainable healthcare that suggest it could have very radical implications for conceptions of good healthcare, more closely corresponding with the potentially 'destabilizing' implications discussed in Section 8.1.

There are tensions and balancing acts both in any attempt to integrate sustainability with other value considerations and in the interpretation of sustainability. We consider these in turn. First, by positing a few illustrative hypothetical questions we explore some value tensions arising from incorporating sustainability as an 'additional' consideration. What if it turned out that the cardiac unit care model showed evidence of being marginally worse in clinical outcomes for a small minority of patients but was still much preferred by patients and substantially better in terms of environmental impact? Assuming that there was no reliable way of identifying in advance which patients would do worse, it could still seem reasonable and defensible to support the change in the light of the considerable benefits to the vast majority of patients, to staff and to the broader good. But this kind of example gives rise to questions such as: how much environmental benefit would need to be demonstrated (and with what certainty) to justify how much loss of clinical benefit (and with what certainty)? How willing would we be to make trade-offs between 'core' aspects of healthcare and (arguably) 'core' social values?

We have argued throughout this book that given the multiple dimensions of and perspectives on quality, balancing acts – for example, between effectiveness and equity – are both inevitable and pervasive. But once we add sustainability into our considerations, conventional healthcare norms can begin to unravel. For example, what if a proposed improvement involved a small loss in clinical outcomes for some reasonably well-served and healthy population but massive reductions in negative environmental impact (with or without financial savings)?

This is analogous to more familiar calls to shift expenditure away from 'low value' healthcare to much more 'productive' uses, perhaps in terms of more cost-effective provision and or better service for poorly served communities and reductions in health inequalities. Given the seriousness of the public health threats from climate change, and especially as what many already describe as a climate emergency becomes more manifest and feels ever more pressing, it is easy to imagine this line of thought being extended. People are already being asked, for the purpose of environmental sustainability, to make adaptations in the ways they buy and use everyday products, heat their homes and travel around. Whole sectors of the economy, including energy production and manufacturing, are reorienting the ways they work. Perhaps one of the adaptations that might now be warranted involves a large-scale disinvestment from many areas of healthcare provision and the encouragement of people to get used to a slimmed down set of services that do most things reasonably well but are also hugely 'greener' and, in that respect, public health oriented?

This line of reasoning returns us to the earlier discussion of rethinking the fundamental bases on which healthcare is judged. Someone with an open-ended concern to improve healthcare and an interest in sustainability might, as just indicated, come to conceive of what improvement entailed, in relation to both ends and means, in markedly different ways to those that currently prevail. People working in the field of healthcare improvement might prefer to limit the potential radicalism of their revisionary perspective and could attempt this in several ways. They might, for example, add sustainability as a secondary 'filter' or discriminator only. As suggested above this would mean first identifying what sets of things would count as quality improvement defined largely in terms other than sustainability (such as clinical effectiveness) and then selecting from various credible options by bearing environmental impacts in mind. The broad defence for this restricting position would be the one already cited – that healthcare represents a distinct set of activities and norms and is at risk of being dissolved unless it is, in some measure, protected from 'colonization' by other agendas. The concern not to sacrifice the needs and interests of current patients for the benefit of future goods and people could also be part of this defence. More pragmatically, people working in healthcare improvement may well feel the need to stick closer to a 'delivery' perspective and (so) to remain strongly connected to the concerns and outlooks of health professional colleagues. Lines could be drawn in this kind of way, but all such attempts would need to be argued for and would be contentious. Boundaries are often unclear: a potentially effective hospital intervention with highly toxic side effects, for example, would be considered questionable on safety grounds. At least to many people, these questions would not magically dissolve if such toxic effects were slower acting and only manifested 'outside' the hospital and managed by a community health team. Services that contribute to a much slower but much broader form of environmental toxicity raise analogous questions. In the end, questions about how to prioritize the various possible constructions of improvement are philosophical and ethical. They might be progressed through deliberation and debate but cannot be settled by fiat.

However, the movement towards including sustainability as a factor in improvement thinking, even when it is interpreted in a contained way as an extra parameter to be borne in mind, is still both relatively radical and, like all other improvement ends, challenging to implement. It requires improvers either to add a further consideration into the mix or, for example, to reconceive existing dimensions of quality such as 'safety' or 'efficiency'. And, even with an emphasis on containing the disruptiveness of the implications, there are considerable uncertainties in determining what improving sustainability entails. Healthcare activities produce carbon emissions but they can affect ecological health in many other ways too – for example, by using other scarce resources including finite supplies (e.g. of certain minerals), by adding to air pollution and water pollution (e.g. though plastics waste), by impacts on biodiversity and animal health, or by negative (or positive) impacts on national or local green spaces and opportunities for experiences of biophilia. When considering environmental impacts, all these merit attention and there is no reason to suppose their implications always point in the same direction. Filtering improvement possibilities using sustainability lenses might easily mean trying to weigh up which of these concerns to prioritize (leaving aside the substantial empirical uncertainty of estimating outcomes given the causal complexities involved). In this regard, sustainability is like the quality concepts discussed in Part 2 – it requires interpretation and contextual application including balancing together multiple implications. There is also the same risk that operationalizations of sustainability obscure its complexity whilst, at the same time, affording greater clarity for measuring and monitoring change. The strong current tendency to equate environmental sustainability in healthcare improvement contexts with the pursuit of net zero carbon emissions undoubtedly supports attention to a major priority, given the grave climate consequences of socially produced 'greenhouse gases', but it is nonetheless a significant simplification.

It is not just at the level of practical application that the idea of sustainability is complex. It is – just like, for example, person-centredness – inherently complex and contested as a concept. Leslie Paul Thiele's overview of the idea of sustainability draws this out very well.[24] Whilst adhering to the broad notion that sustainability is about protecting the long-term viability of activities, and that this involves recognizing deep inter-linkages between the social, economic and environmental conditions of viability, he argues that too much focus can be applied to purely environmental conditions, given that all are needed for sustainability. Greener environmental conditions in the absence of social and economic opportunities do not make for sustainable living conditions and expectations. Thiele argues that addressing sustainability means preserving 'the core functions, values and relationships of the communities of life that sustain us'[25] whilst creatively 'managing the scale and speed of change'[26] such that neither current needs nor future well-being are ignored. Adding the importance of this ongoing cultural creativity to factors alluded to in the 'triple bottom line' of environmental, economic and social goods, Thiele writes:

> [T]o practice sustainability requires us to balance ecological resilience, economic welfare, social equity and cultural creativity. These four goods are compatible and mutually supportive. But that does not mean that all of these goods can be simultaneously maximized. The effort to fully achieve any one of them in isolation will undermine the chances of attaining a good measure of all.[27]

In summary, there are compelling grounds for adding sustainability to the healthcare quality and improvement agenda, and this is becoming accepted. But the inclusion of sustainability as an aim has potential to challenge and destabilize existing improvement norms. Determining how far it is possible and desirable to meaningfully incorporate sustainability within a more conservative delivery framing of healthcare improvement and how far a more revisionary framing is needed to make sense of this inherently long-term, wide-scope value requires philosophical as well as practical deliberation.

8.3 Implementing anti-racism

This section revisits some of the questions raised in the previous two, but with a different example and emphasis. Racism, like environmental sustainability, is a concern that has risen to the top of societal agendas and addressing it is, for good reasons, widely acknowledged to be a moral imperative. There are some parallels with sustainability but also some differences. Racism represents another way in which healthcare can be 'toxic', and it is a phenomenon that is society-wide and not specific to healthcare, albeit not one from which healthcare is exempt. But whereas environmental damage can be seen as a threat and sometimes a cause of subsequent harm to people, racism often operates directly and immediately as well as over time. Racism constitutes moral and practical injury to people and in many instances that damage is instantly manifested. We will return to this idea and its implications for what counts as good healthcare.

Acknowledging and tackling racism might be seen as being implied and perhaps contained within the accepted and standard ambition of healthcare improvement that healthcare should be made 'equitable' – roughly speaking, that the quality of care people get is not a product of (irrelevant aspects of) their personal identity or characteristics.[28] But, as discussed in Chapter 5, ideas such as equity or equality are very broad, contain multiple elements and are open to various interpretations, so it is quite possible for efforts to be directed towards equity without concerns about racism being highlighted. This is especially the case if the covert faces of racism are neglected and where, for example, formal equality of provision is interpreted as a seemingly 'level playing field' of access for all-comers. In policy and professional development discussions, the promotion of anti-racist practices is typically seen as a very important agenda that might have relevance for healthcare improvement but that sits outside the normal confines of the field. We need to ask, then, how might, and how far should, anti-racism be incorporated into healthcare improvement work and what are the challenges and risks of such incorporation?

There can be no serious doubt about whether healthcare embodies racist practices or produces racist effects. It is not part of our ambition to try and map out this critical set of issues, but we can indicate some key aspects of racism as a multi-layered, compound and cumulative phenomenon, and of their challenging implications for improvement work. Tackling racism requires taking into account the effects of history and making use of both public health and interpersonal lenses. One starting point is to recognize that the history of medicine and healthcare includes many examples of 'structural violence' against certain populations and communities. For example, an essay published in *The Lancet* in the wake of the murder of George Floyd in 2020 and in the midst of the COVID-19 pandemic (which was, contemporaneously, highlighting differential health experiences and outcomes) set the ensuing anti-racist protests against a historical backcloth of segregation, exclusion and dramatically unequal patterns of such things as enforced institutionalization, coercive sterilization, experimentation and lack of treatment.[29] The authors underlined that in relation to 'disease intervention in the USA, people of colour have been historically penalized, oppressed and harmed'.[30] Just as with the rest of social life there is no reason to suppose that legacies and patterns of racial discrimination and injustice can be quickly dissolved, or perhaps magically 'switched off'. Indeed, there is plenty of evidence of ongoing racism within healthcare as experienced by both patients and staff members. For example, when surveyed in 2022, a majority of black and minority ethnic leaders working in the UK National Health Service reported having experienced 'verbal abuse or abusive behaviour targeting racial, national or cultural heritage', and from colleagues and managers at least as much as from patients.[31] More than half said they had considered leaving the service because of this treatment and the vast majority lacked confidence in the ability of the organizations they worked for to combat racism and its structural and cultural underpinnings.

Overt forms of racism – whether crude or more subtle – are obviously ethically important because they directly disrespect, demean and undermine people. But they are by no means the only form that racism takes. Racism also takes disguised forms, apparent only in their effects. And whilst the disguise can be deliberate – for instance, where someone self-consciously acts on, but masks, racist attitudes – it need not be. Racism, like other forms of systemic discrimination (e.g. against women), can operate through biases that are built into people's thinking and, crucially, into discursive and institutionalized norms. In other words, healthcare staff can be bound up in racist practices in ways that are not obvious to them. The focus on 'unconscious bias', including the widespread provision of (sometimes mandatory) training about it, is one way services have acknowledged pervasive racism and attempted to respond. But this consideration of individual and group 'psychologies' needs to be set in the context of analogous problems at sociological and system levels. Macro- and micro-conditions that (re)produce racist consequences – such as, on the one hand, unequal educational, employment and housing opportunities and, on the other hand, the effects of implicit biases – interact with institutionalized mechanisms of racism in healthcare, including some built into biomedical knowledge or its usage. These 'meso-level mechanisms' include 'clinical practice guidelines' (CPGs), 'reference value norms' (RVNs) and other standardized protocols or procedures that are often presented, and typically accepted, as 'neutral' but that may reflect various biases and can have unwarranted discriminatory effects.[32] (These concerns about the unintended racist consequences of embedded 'knowledge' have more recently been greatly exacerbated because of the potential power and effects of healthcare artificial intelligence.)[33] Perhaps paradoxically, but significantly, anti-racist efforts to take 'race' into account can also be problematic:

> If race is operationalized in medical guidelines such that racial groups are inappropriately positioned as proxies for assumed differences in physiology, the guidelines themselves can foster inequities across care settings. Specifically, significant equity and justice concerns arise in the development and implementation of CPGs and RVNs that racialize illness thresholds in a way that ultimately requires members of already medically underserved and structurally oppressed racial groups to present with greater illness severity or duration before receiving the same forms of care provided to white patients more readily.[34]

Whatever the exact combination of complex underlying causes, health-related opportunities, policies and practices can embody and/ or produce racial injustices. However unintended these effects are, they are real and ethically serious. For example, as has become well known, Black and Asian women in the UK are far more likely to die in pregnancy or childbirth than white women. There is evidence that their concerns are more likely to be ignored by health professionals, perhaps as a result of racialized stereotypes.[35] Sometimes these racist effects are addressed within the mainstream literature on healthcare quality and improvement with calls for anti-racist responses. For example, a *BMJ Quality & Safety* editorial on diagnostic disparities by Denise Connor and Ghurpreet Dhaliwhal laments that a recent review of studies of responses to patients in US emergency departments showed that Black people were more likely than white people to have cardiovascular diagnoses missed adds to 'the growing evidence base of diagnostic disparities across many clinical conditions such as delayed appendicitis diagnosis in Black children, overdiagnosis of schizophrenia in Black individuals, and delayed dementia diagnosis in Asian and Hispanic/Latinx individuals'.[36] In the remainder of this section, we draw on this editorial, to help explore some of the challenges, including the profound normative complexity, of implementing anti-racism as part of healthcare improvement. Anti-racism has radical implications for improvement work in the sense we rehearsed above, that is, it requires 'deep', as well as 'broad', changes. Addressing racism in healthcare calls for a large range of qualitatively different approaches, both 'top-down' and 'bottom up', and gives rise – as we will elaborate – to risks of being both over-ambitious and under-ambitious and of being counter-productive in multiple ways, potentially leading to harms including further racial injustice.

Anti-racism raises again questions about the appropriate scope of improvement and boundaries between healthcare and public health, and it throws up other deep-seated questions about the conceptual and epistemological framings of improvement agendas. We have already suggested that there might be limits to how far healthcare can 'take on' issues which stem largely from outside the healthcare system, or, at least, how far this is possible whilst maintaining the day-to-day expectations and norms of healthcare. Accepting that those working in healthcare should confront 'healthcare racism' still leaves questions of how far it is appropriate, or even meaningful, for this to be interpreted to include changing broader societal structures except as advocates for, or partners in, such change?

Having noted this problematic, and assuming healthcare actors should be conscientious about anti-racism we come to the need to address conceptual and epistemological frames. Connor and Dhaliwal recognize that '[i]n science, language shapes the research questions we ask, the places we look for solutions and the areas where we invest our resources'[37] and show that this has relevance at various levels. For example, when talking about the effect of 'trust' on people taking up vaccination or treatment options they advocate focusing on institutions that 'lack trustworthiness' rather than individuals who 'lack trust', and avoiding labelling racialized populations as 'high risk' in specific respects but rather recognizing that they are disproportionately subject to structural racism. Such shifts 'switch' the causal lines improvers might focus on and locate the necessity for changes or 'fixes' in the system rather than in the population in question. They include being ready to name 'racism' and include it in the lexicon of improvement rather than relying on 'safer' terms such as equity or inclusion. Amongst other things, Connor and Dhaliwal also highlight the importance of identifying how racial injustices can be 'built into' clinical tools and medical knowledge. Similar analyses are also needed of healthcare improvement knowledge: the danger in all cases is that the frames and power structures embedded in all systems of expertise constrain even the extent to which anti-racist voices and proposals can be heard, let alone enacted. Addressing anti-racism has far-reaching and foundational level implications for improvement. It depends on asking sceptical revisionary questions, not just questions about whether healthcare is being delivered according to its prevailing norms but about the normative constitution of healthcare.

The level of rethinking and re-tooling needed means anti-racism cannot be treated merely as an 'add-on' consideration or easily integrated into mainstream improvement work. Just as with conventional themes in improvement, such as effectiveness and patient safety, it needs some investment of dedicated expertise and reflection. And whilst it overlaps with – that is, has relevance for – these other 'quality dimensions' it is not the same as them. Unless improvers reflect very carefully on the interactions between different dimensions, and the mutual implications of efforts to address them, there is a danger that progress in one area will undermine progress in another without that even being recognized.[38] Anti-racism also calls for both structural and cultural change, both of which can go wrong or, at least, produce contested results. Whilst a broadly public health perspective is essential to identify and attempt to redress unfair distributions in areas like diagnostic validity, access to care and health outcomes, this emphasis on 'outward' measures is not enough. Racism has to be understood, in significant part, as relational and phenomenological. If a person is not 'seen', 'heard' or recognized as an equal by healthcare practitioners because of a racialized identity, then, irrespective of biomedically defined health outcomes, they are badly treated. Care that is shaped to any extent by interpersonal racism is, to that extent, poor care and, indeed, may not be experienced as care at all. Racism in healthcare requires a robust, 'broad-spectrum' response.

As part of proceeding robustly, however, it is essential to be mindful of risks. Along every axis of anti-racist practice there are uncertainties, threats and tensions which we can only summarize here. The use of racialized categories is itself inherently contestable and problematic. It is unsurprising that alongside its reporting experiences of 'Black and Minority' (BME) healthcare leaders (as discussed above), the NHS Confederation, in articulating its anti-racist stance, chooses to highlight the limitations and potential contests around the term BME. This kind of caveat is always relevant and important for any such descriptor and for all systems of 'race' classifications that are used to monitor equity, whether for professionals or patients. Such classifications will inevitably fall short in some respect – they will be too crude to capture all relevant differences or, if they are fine-grained, they will obscure commonalities. And some people may resent being seen through such racialized categories, or feel needlessly 'invisible' or mischaracterized by them. There is no 'happy medium' or clearly right answer here, but pragmatic balances must be found between approaches that provide useful for population insights and to help map potential anti-racist progress and approaches that attempt to recognize and validate the diversity of identities, positions and perspectives.

A similar problem attaches to the effects of making use of such racialized categories. This danger of 'creating new problems' is not specific to the influences of racist assumptions within knowledge-bases and guidance documents but is constantly in play. Using racialized categories always carries the risk of, at least, reifying and reinforcing certain kinds of labels, norms and activities, with potentially racist consequences. Tackling racist attitudes and behaviours is similarly fraught with complications. Especially with unconscious bias, a lot depends upon understanding the perceptions and experiences of both the agent being racist and the person being treated in racist ways. For change to be significant, it needs to be 'absorbed' and accepted by both parties. Clumsy or formulaic interventions can be counterproductive, although, of course, some racist behaviours need to be, and can be, challenged in blunt ways. One illustration of the dangers that accompany well-intentioned efforts comes from education in 'cultural competence' which encourages awareness of cultural diversity and the ways in which values and preference may vary across different groups, but is sometimes enacted or received in ways that can easily serve to reinforce essentializing readings and stereotypes that can themselves be forms of racism.[39]

Another key axis of anti-racist practice is, of course, planning services or improvements with the participation of, or based on co-production with, representatives of those racialized communities experiencing (or likely to experience) racism. Whilst this is unarguably important, the hazards are also well known. There are, for example, dangers of 'tokenism' if the participation is too modest in scope, and, even when the level of joint working is substantial and meaningful, there can be a danger that significant influence and authority is granted to people who are not seen as sufficiently representative or impartial by some sub-populations.

The literature on implementing anti-racist practices in healthcare conveys the level of challenge involved, including some aspects of the problems we have highlighted. For example, following a systematic review of studies of anti-racist training for licensed healthcare professionals, Tiffany Ricks and colleagues concluded: 'A considerable knowledge gap exists regarding effective methods, tools, and outcomes to use for undoing racism' and argued that 'a seismic paradigm shift is called for, one in which an anti-racist perspective informs all healthcare education, research, and practice.'[40] (This suggestion also calls into question the possibility of addressing different improvement aims separately.) The need for a rich, multi-level and multi-component approach is a common theme. This, according to a scoping review of implementing anti-racism interventions in healthcare settings by Nadha Hassen and colleagues, includes dedicated resources, ownership at policy and organizational levels, leadership 'buy-in', including leadership from and partnership with racialized communities, and ongoing staff education and training.[41] The authors also express concern about partial or half-hearted measures, including failures to name racism and an over-emphasis on individual-level educational or language translation initiatives, rather than broader systemic and institutional action. They write:

> Healthcare institutions need to reflect critically on whether they are ready to make the commitment necessary to do this work and invest time and money in the process to bring about sustainable system-level change, or else consider not doing it at all.[42]

One core concern here, reflecting other commentators, is that building any sense of expectation which is then not delivered itself perpetuates racial injustice whilst providing policymakers or institutional leaders with 'moral cover'. Writing about declarations of racism as a public health crisis and the inclusion of Black and Indigenous People of Color (BIPOC) in health strategy making in the United States, Lilliann Paine and colleagues argue:

> Superficial diversity and inclusion efforts that bring BIPOC people and organizers into the conversation and then fail to implement their ideas repeat historical patterns of harm, stall momentum for structural change at best, and poison the strategy at worst.[43]

None of these challenges or complications should discourage action. We rehearse them here to reinforce the point that anti-racist interventions are not something easily designed or incorporated into improvement work. But, more specifically, we want to stress that some of the complexities entailed by aspirations to tackle racism relate to pervasive normative tensions and uncertainties. Unless these are acknowledged and made visible as anti-racist interventions proceed, there is no possibility of even recognizing the range of things that might count as success, let alone achieving them. There is a practical need for philosophical attention to this normative complexity.

8.4 Transforming healthcare

We have looked at environmental sustainability and anti-racism as two important examples of potential changes to healthcare framings and assumptions that carry substantial implications for what counts as 'good healthcare' and hence improvement. These can be seen either as 'new' quality concerns or as part of a fuller unpacking of existing quality concepts. There are, for example, obvious links between environmental sustainability and both 'efficiency' and 'safety', and similar links between 'anti-racism' and both 'equity' and 'person-centredness'. Environmental sustainability and anti-racism are 'radical' in the sense we outlined at the beginning of the chapter in that they relate to basic assumptions or underlying 'roots' of thinking about healthcare purposes and goods.

We can draw out three lessons from the discussion of these examples for healthcare improvement. First, the examples reinforce the key messages of Part 2 of the book that not only is quality plural but so too are the various strands or dimensions of quality: they are each made up of various elements which cannot all be addressed or optimized at the same time. Tensions between elements can arise both 'within dimension' and 'across dimensions' not only because resources (including finances, attention and effort) cannot be used on everything at once and there can be legitimate divergences in what should be prioritized for different parts of a system or from different agent's perspectives, but also because there are practical and conceptual incompatibilities between – or 'contradictory' implications of – elements. Second, these examples further illustrate that there can be no entirely neutral or 'innocent' constructions of improvement. It might make good practical sense for many improvers to focus on small-scale technical improvements in the delivery of specific practices and services but insofar as this means not attending to the less obvious ways in which routine healthcare activities can be toxic, this emphasis and relative neglect embodies a potentially contentious value stance. Third, the examples show how the distinction between the 'depth' and 'breadth' of change – as we hinted earlier – is a blurred one. Although professionals working in a particular unit might usefully be able to conceive of a deep-seated reframing of their work, this rethinking is much less likely to happen and, crucially, is much less likely to result in significant change, if it is not enabled and supported by a parallel change in system norms more broadly.

In concluding we want to say a little about some of the parallels and linkages between 'depth' and 'breadth'. In particular, we consider how the above discussion of 'radical improvement' has relevance for the challenges of healthcare transformation where 'transformation' means bringing about large-scale and sustained change. Specifically, we suggest that our emphasis on the central importance of acknowledging and navigating normative complexity is relevant to the 'scaling up' agenda and resonates closely with emphases found in insightful discussion and scholarship on that theme, albeit that the latter is conducted in genres that are not expressly philosophical.

To begin with, it is worth noting – what should be obvious – that large-scale change is exceptionally difficult to deliberately bring about. (We say 'deliberately bring about' to acknowledge that sometimes large-scale change – for good and/or ill – is 'forced' on systems by historical circumstances including, notably, the recent COVID-19 pandemic.) In addition to the sheer quantity of institutions and actors to be mobilized or steered in various ways, the provision of (some version of) good-quality healthcare has to be maintained throughout – a health system cannot be shut down for ten months while it is redeveloped or replaced (as is sometimes possible with a highway). Despite these inherent and substantial difficulties, there is a tendency for policymakers to attempt to engineer large-scale change with a few simple levers applied from a distance. Indeed, Lorelei Jones and colleagues, who offer a valuable sociological critique of this tendency in the UK NHS,[44] note that '[m]ajor system change retains near mystical attractiveness to politicians and decision makers'.[45] They highlight how such changes cause major disruption and are experienced as troubling by people but typically do not produce the effects intended.

Of particular relevance to the arguments of this book, Jones et al. note the frequency with which the organizational changes they study are based upon top-down, scientistic or algorithmic models, which in turn reflect 'mechanistic rational forms of health service research' or similarly reductionist managerialist conceptions of knowledge.[46] They call for more attention to complexity and ambivalence and the multifaceted healthcare values at stake, including, for example, the ways in which health services carry meanings that transcend their narrow functions and connect to staff and patients' affective lives including their sense of place and trust. There is now a growing body of work that seeks to understand and promote large-scale change whilst, at the same time, moving away from mechanistic top-down thinking. The approach we have encouraged in this book coheres with important strands in this work – in relation to the central importance of learning, dialogue and 'organic' rather than mechanistic thinking. We suggest that the emphasis on normative complexity adds (or at least draws out) something that may be implicit in these promising new emphases but is insufficiently foregrounded.

The Health Foundation, for example, has pulled together insights and resources to support what they consider 'the deep-seated and far-reaching shifts needed in health and care'.[47] Their ambition is that organizational change should not be seen as something 'done to' health services from outside but should be built into the life and culture of healthcare organizations. Central to this ambition are the two linked ideas that (a) thinking about and practising improvement should be mainstream business across all levels of health services and (b) 'learning' matters, in particular that emphasis should be placed on building 'learning health systems'.[48] The thrust of these proposals is, first, that healthcare improvement needs to be thought about not as something that is done by a few 'improvers' in piecemeal and ad hoc ways, but should be embedded everywhere, which means properly resourced, actively involving all staff, patients and communities, and supported by local and national leaders. Second, that part of embedding improvement is that groups of providers, working in conjunction with communities of stakeholders, should be continuously learning about and from the care they provide. This is partly a technical agenda that involves putting in place systems for routinely collecting and analysing data. But it is equally about social and interpersonal adaptation 'to bring people together to ask questions, interpret data, reconcile differing views and make decisions that allows them to successfully effect change in a complex, adaptive system such as health care'.[49]

Chrysanthi Papoutsi and colleagues, in a helpful and theoretically sophisticated overview of approaches to large-scale change, also reinforce the importance of strengthening the system capacity for improvement, and the 'adaptive capability' of staff.[50] This includes investment in human relationships (so people can work together with reciprocity and good will) and the capability to 'productively harness conflict'. Papoutsi and colleagues organize their analysis of 'spread, scale-up and sustainability' by contrast with linear prescriptive models and in recognition of the complexity of health systems, which means that both the knowledge-base for, and practical approaches to, large-scale change must draw on complexity-informed and broader social science perspectives, rather than mechanistic thinking. In relation to the 'scaling-up' of locally successful interventions they note that even relatively successful efforts are often 'a messy process of small wins, compromises, disappointments and deadlocks that do not always lead to the result originally intended'.[51] Working at scale, they underline, should be understood as a phenomenon in its own right and not just as an accumulation of interventions. Because contexts and circumstances vary within health systems, change depends upon what they call 'organic growth' that allows for 'local adaptation, contingency, negotiation, and dialogue'.[52] In short, they argue that because healthcare systems are complex, improvement activities will continuously generate tensions that need to be addressed.

The stress in this literature on learning, dialogue and organic thinking seems very persuasive to us. We additionally want to emphasize the relevance of these themes to understanding and addressing normative complexity, alongside causal or explanatory complexity. Ethical challenges and uncertainties arise not only because circumstances vary, or because of practical obstacles, or because of differences in service histories and trajectories or in professional or personal psychologies, although all of these are significant. Rather, ethical challenges and uncertainties also reflect inherent and pervasive tensions at the core of the healthcare improvement project. And they do not only arise once improvers have decided what matters or counts as 'good' and then face the undoubtedly challenging task of implementation, but rather they also arise in the very process of deciding what matters – a process which runs continuously before, and all the way through and after any implementation.

This normative complexity is very often not acknowledged or brought to the surface. One reason for this, as we noted earlier, is because improvement knowledge is typically couched in technical and relatively value-neutral terms. But, even beyond this fact, it is deeply tempting to resist acknowledging normative complexity. For many practically minded people such an acknowledgement might seem tantamount to stalling progress on the grounds that 'it's all too complicated'. As we have illustrated in this chapter in relation to environmental sustainability and anti-racism (and with respect to other quality concepts in earlier chapters) there are genuinely deep-seated puzzles about how to manage competing considerations when deciding on a way forward. Nonetheless – and we will develop this idea further in the next, concluding, chapter – people do not have the luxury of choosing to *either* act *or* think. It is already a commonplace in many areas – including healthcare improvement – to combine practical action with a parallel process of asking sceptical questions about what is being done. Of course, not everyone has to be doing both things all the time. But, we suggest, in order to 'practise' well it is often valuable (and sometimes necessary) to place normative uncertainties and tensions 'on the table' – and to ensure improvers and institutional stakeholders are alive to and engaged with them.

9 PHILOSOPHY FOR HEALTHCARE IMPROVEMENT

Healthcare improvement, we have argued, is deeply and inevitably bound up with philosophical and ethical questions. This is, in part, in the sense that any social and institutional practice raises philosophical and ethical questions about what people do, how they do it and for what reasons. But healthcare improvement is also specifically concerned with understanding how good things are and with making them better; this raises a set of distinctive questions about what is good and why, and how this can be known and understood. While some of the philosophical and ethical issues raised by improvement are, in some respects, already understood and debated by improvement researchers and practitioners, we have contended that healthcare improvement as a field of practice would be stronger if philosophical reasoning and argument were 'made visible' and allowed to make a fuller contribution to the ideas, discussions, decisions and actions of improvers.

In this final chapter, we summarize and draw together the central themes and ideas that we have introduced and developed throughout the book. Through this, we also say something about how we understand the contribution of the book itself. On the one hand, we have been making a substantive argument about the philosophy and ethics of healthcare improvement, emphasizing the ways in which healthcare improvement is a contested, complex and uncertain space which must be managed through evaluative judgement and open-ended deliberation. While we acknowledge the place for technical schema and measurement within evaluation and deliberation, confining healthcare improvement to these more reductive forms obscures, rather than solves, the normativity, plurality and complexity of improvement practice. On the other hand, we have been making a linked methodological argument about the potential contributions of philosophy to improvement. These two sets of ideas are linked because it is exactly the need for conceptual and ethical open-endedness and interpretation that makes philosophical input particularly valuable – these ways of thinking are philosophy's strong suit. As well as tying together the arguments of the book, in this concluding chapter we say a little more about why philosophers and the tools of philosophy are so well-placed to contribute to improvement. In particular, philosophical reasoning can help to stimulate the more radical and disruptive thinking that is needed for deeper reflection on whether and in what ways the field of improvement is serving healthcare, and the ways in which it may be falling short.

We start in the next section by emphasizing three crucial ideas that we have returned to throughout the book, which are the backbone of our substantive philosophical argument. First, the *implicit normativity* of healthcare improvement research and practice, and the ethical importance of recognizing this and attempting to make implicit value judgements more explicit. Whenever decisions are made about what improvement work to undertake and how, these embody and promote distinctively normative commitments about what matters, the relative priority of different goods and ends, and what health systems and services should be doing and aiming at. Identifying and exploring these commitments helps to expose what and who is being served by existing practice and what and who may be being relatively neglected or wholly overlooked. Second, the conceptual and ethical *pluralism* that characterizes healthcare improvement at all levels, and the value of recognizing and celebrating this, rather than seeing it as a problem to be fixed. Pluralism captures the idea that there are many goods and objects of concern in healthcare improvement and many ways of conceptualizing them. There will rarely be a way of resolving these into a single correct or overarching definition. This is in part because different conceptions are appropriate for different contexts, but also because different people, differently placed, will have different (and often equally valid) perspectives on what is happening, what matters and why. Third, the *normative complexity* of healthcare improvement, which sits alongside explanatory complexity, and introduces uncertainty and interpretability into any claim that something is 'better'. The recognition of normative complexity reinforces concerns about treating improvement as a linear or mechanistic process. It is not merely that potential causal pathways to improvements are difficult to map but also that a judgement that something is 'better' is inherently indeterminate. Normative complexity indicates a substantial role for judgement, deliberation and responsiveness, as well as systems thinking in improvement work. Although these three ideas emphasize the indeterminacy present in healthcare improvement research and practice due to the levels of ambiguity, complexity, uncertainty and contestation present, they need not be seen as unfortunate features which healthcare improvement would be better off without. Rather, they can help make sense of why improvement is so difficult, involving consideration of competing and often incompatible perspectives, trade-offs and risk-taking.

In the following section we then set out the variety of ways in which philosophers and the tools of philosophy can help improvers: the more methodological contribution made by the book. Conceptual analysis can help to identify and interrogate assumptions and concepts that shape and frame improvement practice, and to show when there are alternative ways of looking at the same problems which characterize them differently. Ethical analysis can help to elucidate what matters and why, and to identify and critically assess the values, priorities and goals of different actors and institutions. The tools of practical ethics explore what good decision-making and decision-makers look like in practice and highlight ways in which what seems like a promising idea in theory can be more ambiguous or present ethical dilemmas when enacted or manifested in the real world. Good decision-making might include thinking about the ways that decisions are made, and decision-makers are held accountable, and the degree to which these processes are fair, inclusive and reflect what is important. In all these ways, philosophy can contribute to more robust improvement efforts, insofar as it enables the identification and explicit statement of assumptions and commitments which shape what is taken as valuable and prioritized but would otherwise sit in the background. We have emphasized the ways in which philosophical thinking can highlight the ambiguities, uncertainties and contestation that characterize claims and decision-making about improvement, rather than covering them up or trying to resolve them or explain them away. This demands forms of judgement and interpretation that go beyond consideration of empirical evidence and may present practical challenges for improvers. But it can also strengthen improvement attempts by helping improvers to face the complex and uncertain reality of health systems rather than to artificially simplify and risk misrepresenting them.

In Chapter 8, we suggested that philosophical theories can prompt thinking about more radical change and approaches to improvement and can emphasize ways of thinking about what is good or better that might previously have been neglected or undervalued. Philosophical probing can help to show how the scope of healthcare improvement as a field of practice is bounded by convention and artificially or pragmatically restricted. In this concluding chapter we explore one reason that philosophers are particularly good (though not to the exclusion of others) at this kind of radical and disruptive thinking. Philosophers can play an 'insider-outsider' role with respect to healthcare improvement.[1] They can be insiders insofar as they work closely with improvement practitioners to understand and address the issues which matter to them and try to further the goals of improvement. But, at the same time, they are also outsiders, sitting at a critical distance from the field, which allows them to ask disrupting questions about core or foundational assumptions and conventions, and to question whether the goals of healthcare improvement as currently formulated need to be revisited and changed. Healthcare improvement is a field built on scepticism about whether existing healthcare practices are in fact the best way of doing things, but some of this scepticism is in danger of falling away as improvement becomes institutionalized and formalized. Philosophers can help to keep scepticism alive in improvement, not just because they typically sit outside of healthcare and healthcare improvement institutions, but also because they ask questions and use frames of reference which are outside of normal patterns of thinking among improvers.

Such disruption, used in the right ways, has the potential to strengthen rather than undermine improvement practices, challenging improvers to think about the wider consequences and implications of their work, and giving them the resources to think more clearly and honestly about what is at stake. Embracing the more evaluative side of healthcare improvement – which exists whether it is embraced or not – has the potential to enrich improvement activities and encourage more reflective thinking about the actual and potential social value of healthcare improvement.

9.1 Recurrent themes

In Chapter 1, we set out a philosophical and ethical challenge to claims that are made about improvement: 'but why is that better?' Though we have covered a lot of ground in the intervening chapters, this question has continued to guide our exploration of the issues. We have argued that any claim that some change is for the better, or represents an improvement, will rest on assumptions or commitments about:

- what health systems and services should be doing and how they should be functioning;

- the range of goods and values that healthcare should promote and their appropriate balance and priority;

- what decision-making procedures should be used for planning, delivering, monitoring and evaluating change;

- whose interests healthcare systems should serve and in what ways;

- the appropriate institutional level for delivering different healthcare goods and evaluating healthcare outcomes; and

- what is treated as given and fixed in a healthcare system or service (or in society and social institutions more broadly) and what is up for discussion and change.

As noted above, we have continued to return to three central ideas, which help to make sense of why claims about healthcare improvement are likely to be highly complex, contested and uncertain. In this section, we summarize each idea (implicit normativity, pluralism and normative complexity). We suggest that the complexity and uncertainty that we have exposed should be seen as an asset and not just a burden by improvers. One consequence of improvement being such a contested space is that claims about improvement cannot be taken at face value and require robust and reflective forms of justification.

9.1.1 Implicit normativity

Much of the ethical and conceptual underpinning of improvement claims and activities is implicit. Improvement activities rarely involve overt consideration of their assumptions, especially concerning more foundational ideas about what is good and why, and what the functions of health systems are. In many cases, this is perfectly reasonable – going back to first principles and trying to make each normative and conceptual commitment explicit would result in very few improvement activities getting off the ground. But even if it doesn't always make sense to do deep philosophical analysis, it is important to recognize that these underpinnings are always there, whether interrogated or not. Acting on a claim that something is better – for example, by implementing, scaling up or otherwise endorsing an intervention – will support and validate the implicit values and commitments which underpin it, whether or not this is noticed and whether or not, on reflection, this seems like a good thing.

Stacy Carter describes implicit normativity as the 'unstated or taken-for-granted assumptions about what is good or bad, right or wrong, required or not required' that underpin knowledge claims or other assertions.[2] Throughout the book we have highlighted and drawn out a range of such assumptions in healthcare improvement practice. They include assumptions about the axes or dimensions along which improvement should operate – what improvers should be trying to make better, whether that is the safety of services or how equitable or environmentally sustainable they are – and the relative importance of these dimensions. But they also include assumptions about how improvers should go about finding out what the processes and outcomes of health systems are, when they can be justified in making claims about what is present and absent, and what is better and worse. That is, implicit normativity enters the improvement field via (often uninterrogated) commitments to epistemic norms – about what can be known and how anyone can come to have knowledge and understanding – as well as commitments to substantive ethical norms and values – about what things matter and what is right and wrong. Epistemic norms impact on choices about approaches to improvement and improvement methods, which can themselves impact on more substantive ethical commitments. We have emphasized the ways that certain constructions of healthcare quality, especially ones which emphasize schematic and quantitative ways of describing and coming to understand quality, can preclude meaningful consideration of goods and values which elude measurement and reductive representation. Insistence on 'harder' ways of operationalizing and measuring quality can make it difficult to see the value-laden choices and commitments which are reflected in measures, and the alternative possible ways of understanding and describing what is going on. Factors that cannot be incorporated into such measures can be rendered invisible, and the use of technical operational schema can hide the political and ethical choices which underpin them.[3]

We have also highlighted more structural norms that may shape and constrain improvement activities and the claims that are made about them. These include assumptions about the time frames and institutional boundaries which should be used when measuring and evaluating the impact of improvement projects. How long should improvers wait before saying that they have seen the effects of their interventions? And should they only be looking for effects within their team or institution, or casting the net wider? A narrower frame of reference – temporally, spatially and administratively – will be easier to manage and allow for more definitive answers, but it also has the potential to overlook the ways that health systems interact with other systems and the indistinct boundaries between health outcomes and broader social outcomes. Another set of more structural factors includes conventions around the different roles, responsibilities and activities of different healthcare professionals, including responsibility for decision-making, accountability and ways of communicating. These factors will affect who is involved in decision-making, how different perspectives are incorporated and the ways in which responsibilities and expectations are explicitly or implicitly allocated.

The implicit norms and values that lie beneath often innocent-sounding claims about what is better matter because they affect what improvement activities focus on and what is treated as important. Insofar as people and institutions act on the results of improvement activities, these values are liable to shape what healthcare systems look like, what their goals are and how people think about them. Even if it is not practical to do a philosophical deep dive as part of every improvement project, it may be important to always include some reflection on the underlying assumptions about what matters, what is good or bad and what is treated as given. Making some of the implicit normativity more explicit generates opportunity to reflect on whether assumptions are well founded and whether other values are being systematically overlooked or underplayed. Occasionally, it will be important for those with more managerial or executive roles to initiate conversations about some of the more foundational questions about system goals and institutional boundaries. Sometimes reflection on norms will identify problems with dominant framings which will generate shifts in values. But even when, on reflection, improvers decide that they were operating with a well-founded set of norms and assumptions, the process of reflection can help them to construct strong justifications for their claims and decisions.

9.1.2 Pluralism

At its most general, pluralism is the idea that there are two or more entities or processes, which can't be reduced to one another or some third thing. We have argued that quality is plural. This is not just in the widely acknowledged sense that there are many dimensions of quality, but also in two further senses: first, that there are different, irreducible ways of defining and characterizing quality which are appropriate for different settings or in support of different purposes.[4] There is no way of resolving these different conceptions of healthcare quality into a single, universal definition or framework. Second, even if an appropriate definition of quality has been selected for a given purpose, there will be different ways of operationalizing this, through using different indicators, measures and datasets. These forms of plurality mean that, if a quality framing is to be used in improvement activities, pragmatic choices must be made between different quality conceptions and different operational definitions. It is not just the high-level definition of quality that is plural, but its constituent parts too – there are many different, irreconcilable ways of understanding what it is for care to be 'safe', 'person-centred', 'sustainable' or whatever other quality attributes are sought. We have also indicated that 'quality' framings are just one way of characterizing healthcare for the purpose of improvement, so pluralism in healthcare improvement extends beyond thinking about healthcare quality and is a more general feature of the concepts, values and goods relevant to thinking about improvement.

Working out how best to define or characterize healthcare for improvement purposes will involve deliberation about the purposes for which a system is being assessed and the specific context in which it is to be evaluated. There will be many ways of understanding and particularizing what is good, which generate different improvement claims, and the resulting patchwork adds further contestability into claims about quality and improvement. This plurality also means that caution must be exerted when transposing models of quality and claims about improvement from one setting to another. We highlighted the ways in which definitions of quality and its dimensions, and assessments of quality and improvement, are contextual and linked to particular purposes. While there may be reasons to make more general claims about healthcare services which can be compared across different settings, these are liable to be of limited use if we want to understand the functioning and value of specific services.

One important upshot of pluralism is that any given definition or measure of healthcare quality – or improvement-related values – is not usefully understood as definitively characterizing or measuring its object. Rather, these tools can help improvers to describe and understand healthcare practice, but they do so in limited ways, capturing only some of the things of value that are promoted by and reflected in healthcare. Definitions and measures of healthcare goods and values should be seen as partial and defeasible, needing to be used in combination with other measures and sources of information, rather than giving clear and final answers about how good healthcare services are. While this certainly adds a good deal of variability and contestation to the field and practice of improvement, we think that recognizing pluralism has the potential to add significant richness and depth. For it suggests that the best way of evidencing claims about improvement is not to spend a lot of time determining exactly the right things to measure and ways of measuring them, but rather to investigate and measure a range of things related to the object of interest – be that safety, person-centredness, effectiveness or any other healthcare value – using a range of different sources and methods that will together start to build a nuanced picture of practice. One consequence of this is that there are unlikely to be clear and precise answers coming out of the resulting patchwork of measures and evidence. This does not mean that the information they provide is not useful, nor that it is not accurate. But it does mean that deliberation, judgement and more holistic forms of evaluation are needed to determine how to understand and act on the array of data.

9.1.3 Normative complexity

In some respects, the complexity of health systems is increasingly well accepted and understood. Complex systems are unpredictable in detail, which makes it difficult to say with certainty what the outcomes of any given intervention will be, though they do exhibit patterns and forms of equilibrium.[5] Small changes can have large effects, or effects in parts of the system to which they are not obviously or directly connected; system processes are affected by 'external' as well as 'internal' factors. For improvers, this means that predictions and claims about the causal efficacy of improvement interventions are riddled with uncertainty and cannot be assumed to apply in new contexts. We have introduced the idea of *normative complexity*, which co-exists with this causal complexity but has been less well considered. Normative complexity captures the idea that in a complex system, it is difficult to say with certainty whether some intervention or change will make things better, and what its ethical impact will be.

Healthcare systems exhibit normative complexity, as we have described it, in various ways, many of which relate to their causal complexity. Here we highlight three, all of which are closely connected with the forms of pluralism just discussed. One aspect of normative complexity is that healthcare systems comprise many different interconnecting subsystems, serve a variety of different functions and can be judged good or bad in many different ways. This means that any claim that some intervention or practice is 'good' or 'better' is unlikely to be straightforwardly or obviously true: while it may improve things in some ways or generate benefits of some kinds, it will also have opportunity costs which mean that resources are diverted from other goods or goals. It may also have downsides which undermine one or more important healthcare functions at the same time as it furthers and promotes others. Claims about good or better healthcare thus involve evaluative judgements which weigh up multiple factors, assessing their relative priority. At different times, or in different parts of the system, a similar situation might well merit a different judgement about what is good and better.

A second aspect of normative complexity is connected to the fact that many different people interact with healthcare systems, designing and planning them, executing their core and more peripheral functions, and using their services – and often engaging in more than one of these roles at the same time. Different people, differently placed, have different perspectives on what a health system is doing and how well it is functioning. This is in part because people see and experience the system differently, but also because they have different preferences, values and interests relating to it. No one perspective is correct or otherwise inherently better than others, because they reflect different normative perspectives on a system which does many things for different people. But such an array of perspectives can result in disagreements about what is good or better, and there are limited ways of resolving or adjudicating between such disagreements because there is no neutral position from which to judge them.

A third aspect of normative complexity emerges because the boundaries between what is internal and external to the healthcare system are indistinct. Healthcare systems are deeply intertwined with other social systems. For example, the health and health prospects of people entering the healthcare system – where that is understood in terms of formal healthcare institutions – are affected by social and environmental factors usually treated as external to healthcare, such as income and wealth, ethnicity and cultural background, and geographic location. The activities that go on within healthcare systems also impact on things other than health, such as people's income and wealth, ability to work and perform day-to-day activities, and their well-being or life satisfaction more generally. And, to take another example, the functioning of healthcare systems is affected by the broader economic and political environment, which will shape funding, workforce, equipment and other resources such as pharmaceutical therapies and other therapeutic tools. The way healthcare systems are run also has potential to affect economics and politics in turn, not least because they are typically nationally significant employers. Judgements about what is good and better can be made with a different scope in mind – what is better in institutional terms, or thinking about the long-term interests of patients, or thinking about broader social or political or environmental factors – and these need not align.

All these aspects of normative complexity occur simultaneously and interact with one another, and together they introduce very high levels of uncertainty and interpretability into any claim that some intervention or practice is good or better than others. Better in what ways? Better according to whom? Better for what? This need not result in total paralysis or prevent any justified claims from being made about improvement, but it does mean that judgement, deliberation, conversation and more open-ended forms of reasoning and decision-making need to play a central role in any improvement activities. It also indicates that claims that are made about improvement, and decisions and actions taken on the basis of them, will likely reflect some ideas about what is better and the values of some people or institutions but not others. We suggest that improvers should adopt an attitude of humility and continual awareness of the limitations of their improvement claims and knowledge, just as they customarily view their causal claims and knowledge as defeasible and to some extent uncertain.

9.1.4 Normativity, pluralism and complexity as assets

These three ideas – implicit normativity, pluralism and normative complexity – are closely related. All of them stem from the fact that healthcare improvement is a value-laden practice, which reflects what is deemed to be good and bad healthcare as much as it reflects empirical evidence about what healthcare practice is and isn't doing and achieving. All of them point to high levels of contestation and uncertainty in improvement claims and improvement activities. Many improvers might consider this an unfortunate feature of healthcare improvement and would like to reduce or eliminate the disagreement and ambiguity in claims about healthcare quality and improvement.

Resolving disagreement and uncertainty is, to some extent, necessary for successful healthcare improvement in practice, but we think there is good reason to acknowledge and even celebrate these features. One simple but important reason is that disagreement and uncertainty exist in healthcare and healthcare improvement, and to act as if they don't risks endorsing claims and decisions that do not reflect the realities of practice. Healthcare improvement does not just assess the state of healthcare but is used to design and justify changes intended to make healthcare better. Improvement recommendations that are based on an inaccurate or simplistic picture of healthcare systems and values are liable to create problems because they overlook important activities and goods which are in fact necessary for good functioning of the system. Recognizing the uncertainty and disagreement that characterize and underlie healthcare improvement activities may also make a practical difference to those involved in or affected by improvement activities. If those who lead or promote improvement activities insist that the recommended actions definitively and exhaustively reflect what is good, then those who disagree, or who see the significance of other values which are not captured in the recommendations, may feel that their perspectives and interests are being disregarded. Alternatively, improvement leaders could acknowledge the contestation involved in making improvement claims and decisions and the trade-offs and pragmatic decisions that are required to pursue healthcare improvement in practice. This might, for example, involve encouraging more explicit conversations about the ways in which pursuing some aims entails paying less attention to other important aims, at least in the short term, and how attention to certain values promotes the interests of some groups of people over others. As part of this, improvers might be encouraged and enabled to make more explicit statements about the trade-offs they are considering and making. While such statements would not themselves change the recommendations or actions, they would signal to stakeholders that their interests and perspectives are not being overlooked. Such an approach might also help to ensure that a range of perspectives are reflected in improvement activities in the longer term, even if not all perspectives can be reflected in every project or decision.

Attention to disagreement, uncertainty and trade-offs can help to explain why improvement is so difficult, not just in the sense that it is difficult to make changes which clearly demonstrate improvement, but also in the sense that it is psychologically difficult for improvers to manage trade-offs and tension, risks and responsibilities, conflict and factions, and the indefinitely large amounts of evidence and potential evidence that characterize healthcare improvement activities. Rather than giving the impression that improvement should be relatively straightforward, recognition of its challenges may be an important way of supporting improvers and those impacted by improvement activities to continue with their work without feeling threatened by decisions or anxious about their own capacities.

9.2 Contributions of philosophy to healthcare improvement

These more substantive arguments about healthcare improvement indicate an ongoing role for philosophical thinking in improvement practice. All improvement decisions involve evaluative judgement and interpretation and, at least sometimes, improvement practice requires more wide-reaching ethical deliberation about what healthcare systems should be doing and why. This is not to say that professional *philosophers* are always needed to do this philosophical thinking, although their input might sometimes be valuable as we will discuss in the following section. In this section, we review and summarize some of the ways that philosophical thinking can contribute to healthcare improvement.

One philosophical tool that is crucial to sufficiently nuanced and reflective improvement work is conceptual analysis. To explain the importance and role of conceptual analysis, Mary Midgley compares philosophy with plumbing:

Plumbing and philosophy are both activities that arise because elaborate cultures like ours have, beneath their surface, a fairly complex system which is usually unnoticed, but which sometimes goes wrong. In both cases, this can have serious consequences. Each system … is hard to repair when it does go wrong, because neither of them was ever conspicuously planned as a whole.[6]

However, Midgley notes, unlike with plumbing, where the need for specialist intervention to identify and fix problems is well accepted, in the case of philosophy people 'not only doubt the need, they are often sceptical about whether the underlying system even exists at all'.[7] The consequences of misfunctioning and disordered concepts are less obvious than a drip coming through a light fixture or a flooded back yard: instead, they 'quietly distort and obstruct our thinking'.[8] Philosophy, Midgley suggests, can help us to readjust our concepts by identifying and shifting the set of assumptions that we have inherited, and which shape our thought. In this task, philosophical thinking must play a difficult balancing act between setting out a new vision and carefully articulating the details and consequences of the new scheme. While some of this work can be carried out by any critically reflective actor, where more substantial conceptual problems are concerned, concerted theoretical and conceptual analysis will be necessary – at least sometimes involving professional philosophers.

A concrete example will help bring this to life. We have returned a few times through the book to the shift from a 'Safety-I' to 'Safety-II' conception of patient safety, a prominent conceptual shift in healthcare improvement. Safety-I is a conceptual scheme which characterizes safety in terms of what goes wrong. Safety, on this view, amounts to the avoidance of preventable iatrogenic harm where, on the whole, things go wrong because of identifiable failures or malfunctions of specific components, such as technology, procedures, workers or institutions.[9] According to this conceptualization of safety, improving the safety of patients involves methods such as reducing variation in performance and outcomes, using checklists and standard operating procedures, and careful investigation to determine the source of the error when things have gone wrong. However, Safety-I approaches can create problems. A focus on what goes wrong can justify blaming and punishing individuals when things go wrong if the harm can be attributed to a particular decision or (in)action. In practice, such a convention can drive people to cover up their behaviour, not report harmful or adverse events, or find ways to pass the blame onto others. A culture of blame which emphasizes wrongdoing might also encourage healthcare professionals to work strictly to contract, ensuring that they are always legally in the right to protect themselves, even if this involves behaving in ways which do not serve patients well. Safety-I is also connected to the publication of rankings of healthcare professionals. In the UK, published surgical outcomes data allows colleagues, journalists and the general public to see the risk-adjusted mortality rates for each named consultant surgeon in a range of surgical specialities.[10] 'Outliers' are investigated, and sometimes disciplinary action is taken. While there are benefits to such practices, which may be thought to increase transparency for patients and commissioners, empower them as decision-makers and provide a good measure of clinical effectiveness, they can also have negative effects. For instance, if a whole team is involved in any surgery, supported by a much larger set of institutional systems and practices, but only the consultant's name is associated with outcomes, surgeons may be incentivized to prevent trainees from being involved in higher-risk or more complex cases.[11] Although this would avoid the risk of trainees making a mistake or performing tasks less skilfully than consultants might themselves, it also has the potential to deny trainees the experience they need to become skilled and practised surgeons. Consultant surgeons themselves may also be less inclined to take on more complex cases.

One way of thinking about what is going wrong here is that at the root of these problems is a badly functioning conceptual scheme. Well-meaning efforts to reduce the amount of harm and ill health caused by healthcare and within healthcare institutions can incentivize behaviours that are dysfunctional and sometimes end up undermining the safety and health of patients. Safety-II is a different conceptual scheme, which emphasizes what is going on when things go right, and the huge role that responsiveness and adaptiveness to changing conditions play in effective healthcare is a philosophical solution to these problems. It represents a shift in thinking about safety with implications for healthcare practices and behaviours. Notably, the conceptual shift to Safety-II enables improvers to see the healthcare landscape through a different lens, showing factors to be relevant to safety which were previously seen as irrelevant. We are not trying to suggest that the conceptual framing of Safety-I is the only cause of the problems associated with some efforts to improve safety, or that these problems are inevitable. Rather, we want to emphasize how the ways concepts are framed and understood can shape and drive behaviour because they bring different values and objects into focus as salient and important and put others out of focus.

The shift to Safety-II is an example of a deep and fairly radical conceptual shift. Much of the conceptual analysis that could be helpful to improvers and improvement practice is far less radical and does not require formal theoretical analysis to explain and justify it. For example, people involved in an improvement project in an acute hospital setting might reflect on how they conceptualize clinical effectiveness and realize that they are using only short-term endpoints for measuring outcomes. Considering longer-term endpoints, and perhaps looking at measures of quality of life and experience as well as mortality and readmission rates, could give different – and almost certainly richer – pictures of effectiveness. This constitutes a reconceptualization of effectiveness and involves a conceptual shift, albeit in a limited way. Such a shift might lean on existing theoretical literature and discourse which highlight the limitations of narrowly clinical understandings of effectiveness in improvement, but it need not entail any larger institutional or systemic changes in how the concept and language of effectiveness is used: it is quite possible for a single improvement project to rethink some of its concepts without this having broader systemic ramifications. Nonetheless, such reflection involves philosophical reasoning and conceptual analysis akin to what goes on in more radical conceptual tinkering – it is analytical work of a different degree rather than a different kind. Though we have not necessarily used this label, we have been discussing conceptual analysis throughout the book, when exploring how quality concepts are defined and operationalized, how the scope and timescales of improvement are conceived, and the presence and role of more delivery and revisionary perspectives in the improvement field. We have emphasized the value of reflection on how the concepts that are used by improvers and the ways they are understood affect the decisions and actions that are taken in improvement work, and what it would look like to place emphasis on altered or altogether different concepts. This work is valuable because conceptual schemes can powerfully shape and constrain action, but also because dominant or embedded concepts rarely reflect the only way of understanding what healthcare systems do and should do, and how they could be better.

It is worth noting that this conceptual work can be explicitly ethical, when the concepts under consideration are distinctively ethical ones like equality, care, kindness, trust and so on. Such work can also concern categories that are more ontological or epistemological – about what exists and what we can know – as might be the case if questions arise about different ways of conceptualizing and understanding the relationship between an intervention and context, or how to define what the consequences of an action are and where to draw the lines around what is counted and what is not. Even if not obviously ethical issues, these do have normative implications, insofar as they are used to characterize what are treated as improvement aims and what is treated as important. And when such definitions are used to shape decisions and actions, they have concrete effects in healthcare systems, shaping what does and doesn't get done and often whose interests are served and whose are not.

As well as conceptual ethical work, other forms of ethical reasoning play a crucial role in improvement. One idea that we have returned to throughout the book is how balancing and making trade-offs between different aims, values and goods are central to improvement work. This process involves assigning relative priority to different goods – where this priority may be specific to a particular point in time or a particular issue – and determining what balance of them to promote and pursue. This work remains to be done after conceptual issues have been settled, because conceptual analysis will leave a number of important aims and values in place, which improvers will need to work out how to manage in relation to one another. Even if there is agreement about what values and goods are important and their broad definition, different ways of prioritizing them and trading them off against one another will result in quite different consequences. We have highlighted how improvement values and goods will relate to one another in complex ways – sometimes mutually supportive and sometimes conflicting – and how it is unlikely to ever be possible to pursue every desirable end at once. Complicating this picture is the different emphasis and priority given to different aims and values by different people and groups, such that different trade-offs will serve their interests and perceived interests differently.

In bioethics there is a strong theoretical tradition of decision-making in the face of reasonable pluralism where that includes both pluralism in the sense of there being many different values, and pluralism in the sense of there being many different ways of conceptualizing those values. Perhaps the best-known example of this is Tom Beauchamp and James Childress' 'principlism', which proposes that four core values lie at the centre of all healthcare decisions: respect for autonomy, beneficence (doing good), non-maleficence (avoiding harm) and justice.[12] We are not principlists, and we think there is much more at stake in healthcare decision-making than these four values. However, we think that Beauchamp and Childress are right to stress the idea that there are a range of conflicting and interacting values in healthcare, and decision-making involves contextual balancing and making trade-offs between these. In other words we endorse approaches to bioethics that embody value pluralism, whether that is within principlism or more case-based approaches.[13] Case-based or casuistic approaches emphasize the importance of comparing and contrasting particular cases, rather than appealing to pre-determined moral principles, in moral decision-making. Case-based approaches typically emphasize that very little can be said about the relevance or weight of any moral principles or theories to practical decision-making without first considering the concrete particulars of cases. Whereas principlism sees reflection on principles as helping to determine what to do in particular cases, case-based accounts see reflection on particular cases as helping to determine what moral principles there are and how they might apply in practice.

We doubt that decision-makers in practical settings, acting ethically, use any clearly defined method of moral reasoning, although consideration of both specific cases and more general principles do seem like useful tools in reflecting and deliberating about what is good and why. And moral reasoning will not necessarily be improved by use of any particular philosophically sanctioned method. Perhaps more important is the process of deliberation itself. We have emphasized deliberation as a form or part of decision-making which involves open-ended reflection on a range of different issues and options to come to an overall holistic judgement about a question that doesn't have a straightforward answer. Whatever ethical balancing looks like in practice, the forms of pluralism we have discussed and the indeterminacy about the best way to characterize a range of goods and values relating to healthcare and improvement make deliberation indispensable for anyone trying to make nuanced and sensitive decisions about trade-offs. We have emphasized that the use of harder measures of healthcare quality and other values does not obviate the need for deliberation, as such measures will rarely if ever give a definitive answer on how systems are functioning or whether a change is an improvement. This is not just because such measures sit alongside other actual and potential evidence and measures, which may take different forms and not be directly comparable, but also because constructing any measures involves a series of non-trivial evaluative judgements. Deliberative dialogues and conversations are central to managing the complexity and pluralism that characterizes healthcare improvement decisions, because these are communicative forms which allow for consideration of different perspectives, take disagreement and difference seriously and can hold complexity. When used as a decision-making tool, deliberation can be used to try to find common ground and routes to practical solutions which adequately account for the range of factors and views at stake and which appropriately balance important goods.

Alongside deliberation, we have highlighted other forms of practical ethics which are central to reflective healthcare improvement practice, including the development of virtues among healthcare professionals and leaders. Virtues go beyond technical knowledge and skills and reflect the full range of professional and human values which are needed for ethically sensitive improvement work. We have also discussed the importance of listening to and including a range of voices in decision-making, to reflect the variety of different perspectives on and experiences of healthcare. These tools of practical ethics aim at good context-sensitive decision-making – recognizing that well thought-through theories about what is good and better can fall apart when they meet the realities of healthcare practice: operating at scale, across time and space, accommodating human psychology and difference, and contending with existing systems and practices. We have emphasized that ethical practice requires much more than a worked-out theory of *what* is right and good – it also involves thinking about *how* to bring desirable goods and values to life. One important component of this is that many important values such as fairness, equity, person-centredness and respect do not just describe desirable end-states that health systems should be aiming at but also describe valued ways of getting there. The *means* of improving healthcare – where that includes the way decisions are made, the way staff and patients are treated and the way that practical and ethical capability is developed – are just as much a part of 'good' healthcare as the ends that are sought.

There are, then, a number of different ways in which philosophical approaches and reasoning can serve improvement. These are tools which can be, and often already are, used by improvers – you don't need to be a professional philosopher to do conceptual analysis or practical ethics. Reflecting and deliberating on conceptual and ethical issues are activities that are continuous with good, ordinary practical decision-making. But we have suggested that more explicit attention to the normativity of practical decision-making, the conceptual pluralism which characterizes the improvement landscape and the ethical implications of improvement decisions can add another layer to reflective improvement practice and make improvement decisions more robust and accountable insofar as they better reflect the complexity and contestation at stake. Improvement demands forms of judgement and interpretation that go beyond the production and consideration of empirical evidence. Recognizing the normativity and pluralism which characterizes all improvement activity may seem like a problem and a burden for improvers, but trying to manage the indeterminacy and contestation that it generates by using only technical decision-making tools and fixed and closed definitions, specifications and measures will hinder rather than help. For this will merely hide, rather than resolve, the complexity, and potentially creates big problems in the long term, even if it creates the appearance of success in the short term.

This is not to say that it will be appropriate for everyone involved in improvement to be considering all this plurality and uncertainty and normativity at all times. While some such consideration and deliberation may appropriately be part of every improvement project, there will be some topics that are best reflected on occasionally rather than continually, and other topics that may be best considered at a policy or leadership level rather than by everyone involved in improvement. For example, it could be extremely valuable for an institution to have oversight of its improvement projects to ensure that there are not conflicts between them, and to ensure that important values are being served and promoted across the range of projects, even if not every project focuses on every important value at once. But it would be unreasonable and inefficient to demand that this synoptic work be performed by all improvers: such work requires an overview which will often only be available to people in systems or institutional leadership positions. And, rather than expecting each improvement project to determine how to define and measure complex social goods – like communication, patient and staff needs and experience, and equality – institutions could hold occasional deliberative events to discuss how best to understand and capture them, allowing for open and inclusive discussion of challenging and contested questions and ensuring that a range of perspectives are heard and some of the complexity involved is reflected. In practice, incorporating philosophical thinking into improvement requires attention to the variety of roles played by healthcare practitioners and their differing institutional and social locations and perspectives. This responsiveness includes realistic consideration of the capacity for different kinds of decision-making and reflection that are afforded by their respective positions.

9.3 Distinctive role of philosophers

Alongside the extensive practical philosophy that we are suggesting should be part of improvement efforts and employed by improvement practitioners and researchers, there may also be a distinctive role to be played by philosophers, who typically sit outside of healthcare institutions and are well-situated to pose more foundational challenges to improvers. By 'philosophers' here we mean those people who are in a position to engage in philosophical thinking in a concerted manner and in a sustained way over time – this often means professional philosophers but includes others with relevant training, interests and dispositions. In this section, we discuss what philosophers can bring to the table. Midgely notes that it can be helpful for trained philosophers to contribute to conceptual analysis because they bring relevant knowledge of conceptual problems in other areas, and understand how conceptual developments have worked elsewhere. They also tend to have a useful set of skills, combining 'both the new vision that points the way we are to go and the logical doggedness that sorts out just what is, and what is not, involved in going there'.[14] This suggests that input from philosophers might be especially valuable when tackling a particularly tricky or substantial conceptual or ethical issue, and for helping others to learn how to think more philosophically. While this may be true, we want to emphasize other roles for philosophers that we think are also important within the improvement context, because they can less easily be played by dedicated improvers. Again 'philosophers' here certainly includes people employed as professional philosophers but, fundamentally, refers to those who are drawn to and invested in philosophical work and thinking. As the discussion of Safety-I and Safety-II in Section 9.2 illustrated, philosophical contributions can be made by people working under different disciplinary labels and there will be some significant overlaps between contributions from philosophers and those who are pressing and tackling foundational questions from other disciplinary traditions.

In Chapter 8, we indicated the disruptive potential of philosophers to pose radical challenges and reframe healthcare and improvement in ways which unsettle the status quo. This might involve asking open-ended questions about what healthcare is for and what the function of healthcare institutions is, and perhaps identifying values and goods which have been overlooked, deprioritized, or acknowledged and promoted only in shallow and inadequate ways. Certain questions may sometimes be difficult for improvers to hear because they critically interrogate longstanding conventions and central assumptions, or methods, or institutional or disciplinary boundaries that are central to how improvers understand their own professional identity and their work. Such radical interventions will not necessarily lead to epiphanies and drastic shifts in behaviour or thinking – indeed they are perhaps more likely to meet resistance – but they can be part of ongoing reflection on the norms of healthcare and healthcare improvement practice and so contribute to changes in the way people think and work. The examples of sustainability and anti-racism that we explored in Chapter 8 are instances of current debates connected to changing norms and social values. The idea of person-centredness is a good example of a conceptual and practical shift which has moved into the mainstream; it may not yet be a new norm, but it is probably no longer best described as a 'radical' idea. Some important radical questions have yet to be considered in a sustained way – such as how far the locus of improvement can or should semi-detach itself from either biomedical or managerial frames (important though these frames are), why healthcare improvement doesn't engage more with public health, and how a shift from 'healthcare' improvement to 'health' improvement might transform the field.

Philosophers, we think, are well-disposed and well-placed to make such challenges. Here we highlight two reasons for this: first, because typically philosophers operate with a good deal of methodological flexibility, they can inhabit a kind of 'trickster' role, questioning and redrawing established boundaries and revealing ways in which fundamental assumptions can be exposed and transformed. Second, because philosophers tend to operate professionally at some distance from the field of healthcare improvement, as interlocutors they can adopt an 'insider-outsider' stance, where they are responsive and attentive to the existing goals of improvement practice but also maintain a critical attitude towards them. These two roles enable philosophers to make a distinctively sceptical contribution to improvement, which supports the more familiar forms of scepticism that are already central to improvement activities and research.

9.3.1 Scepticism and philosophers as tricksters

Philosophy is characterized by an unusual methodological openness, which enables philosophers to be distinctively unrestricted in terms of the kinds of questions they ask and the kinds of answers they give. There is a strong philosophical tradition of methodological critique – challenging the methods and structures used in the sciences and social sciences in particular and exploring the limits of their claims to knowledge and understanding. But philosophers do not necessarily operate with an explicit or clearly defined method themselves, using a range of different argumentative and deliberative tactics to question and examine ways of talking, thinking, doing and being. One key component of philosophical reasoning is *scepticism*, that is, the use of targeted and sometimes systematic doubt to test knowledge and beliefs in efforts to acquire truth and certainty, even if that is just certainty about what is unknown. While radical scepticism – doubting that anything can be known – is part of some philosophers' practice, we think that more localized and pragmatic forms of scepticism equip philosophers for meaningful and valuable contributions to social practices such as healthcare improvement. That is, they can use targeted scepticism to help practitioners think about what is valuable and important, and the extent to which this is reflected in and promoted by their work. The idea is not to undermine healthcare improvement activities, but to stimulate practitioners to think about the assumptions and conventions which are involved, and to explore whether any of them should be overturned or modified. Philosophers working in applied settings might look at some group of practitioners and ask: 'What kinds of things are they talking about?' or 'What kinds of things are they doing?' and then: 'Are there different or better ways of characterizing this?'[15] New characterizations may sometimes diverge from the ways that practitioners describe and understand their own work. This is a kind of sceptical conceptual analysis, where the way that concepts are being used is subjected to critical scrutiny. But it is quite methodologically open because there is not a pre-determined framework which specifies what form answers can take, and ideas are subject to scrutiny from within a very wide-ranging scope.

Scepticism is a key element of science and social science too – scientists suspend judgement, even about things that may appear obvious, until they have evidence which amounts to a conclusive proof or explanation. Indeed, healthcare improvement is a field built on scepticism: questioning and examining the value and implications of normal and entrenched healthcare practice are a central part of improvement activities, with improvers maintaining scepticism about 'what works' until satisfactory evidence can be produced. Philosophical scepticism is similarly concerned with doubting and examining embedded assumptions, but it operates with a very broad scope. Philosophical scepticism extends not just to questioning the knowledge claims within disciplines and the methods used to arrive at them but also to challenging the conceptual and ethical assumptions that underpin and characterize the questions that are asked and the answers that are given. When faced with a question like 'Does x improve healthcare quality?' philosophers are unlikely to settle on a yes or no answer without first asking basic but searching questions like 'what is quality?', 'what are the aims of healthcare?', 'what would count as improvement?', '(why) should we by trying to improve healthcare quality?', 'is it ethical to do x?', 'is x important or the kind of thing we should be focusing our attention on anyway?' and so on. In other words, if you ask a philosopher a question you might not get the answer you were looking for!

When philosophers play this part, they can be thought to be inhabiting a 'trickster' role. A trickster is an ambiguous figure in myth and folklore who subverts and questions the status quo. Tricksters can act in foolish or subversive ways, but often in so doing transcend the social order and make social hierarchies and restrictions look silly or arbitrary. Lewis Hyde emphasizes their status as 'boundary-crossers'.[16] Sometimes tricksters are portrayed as literal shapeshifters, like Loki in Norse mythology. At other times they more metaphorically cross boundaries, mediating between people and contexts or acting as messengers, like Prometheus in Greek mythology or Coyote in Native American mythology. This may involve dissolving boundaries or showing them to be ambiguous, and sometimes it involves redrawing boundaries or disclosing previously hidden distinctions.[17] Helen Lock notes similarities between the trickster and the fool – a character who can appear foolish but reveal unpleasant or awkward truths, and can be wise because they say what they see rather than adhering to conventions and acquiescing to authority:

> For the fool, as for the trickster, boundaries are not so much nonexistent as arbitrary (new or different boundaries can be created at will), and the comic play of his folly lies in his refusal to accept or recognize what seems self-evident to those who govern boundaries.[18]

Seeing philosophers as tricksters draws out some important characteristics of their methods and approaches. Rather than operating with a clear and distinct framework for knowledge creation, philosophers can 'increase the sphere of hermeneutical possibilities,'[19] that is, increase understanding by exposing and exploring different interpretations of what is said and done. This hermeneutic expansiveness is echoed in the pluralism and high degree of interpretability that we have argued are central to healthcare improvement. And the trickster's ability to reveal hidden or unacknowledged assumptions is echoed in our arguments about the implicit normativity of improvement. Like tricksters, philosophers adopt, and can encourage others to adopt, questioning, critical attitudes towards the world, not taking things at face value, and challenging established concepts, categories, norms and institutions. In the context of improvement, this might involve asking questions that are counter-cultural and difficult to entertain because they call fundamental tenets of the field into doubt. But, when well formulated, such questions can expose unfounded assumptions and conceptual lacunas which are not typically noticed because they are so deeply integrated in normal practice. Lock articulates the power of such tactics: 'The true trickster's trickery calls into question fundamental assumptions about the way the world is organized, and reveals the possibility of transforming them.'[20] Similarly, we see a role for philosophers not just as interminable critics, but as playing a more constructive, positive role in exposing the possibility of other ways of doing and thinking about improvement.

9.3.2 Philosophers as insider-outsiders

A second set of characteristics make philosophers especially well-suited to asking subversive and potentially destabilizing questions. Philosophers can adopt an 'insider-outsider' stance, wherein they are both responsive and attentive to the goals and practices of improvers and, at the same time, freed from certain disciplinary norms and constraints, enabling them to adopt a more critical and revisionary perspective.[21] Philosophers who seek to feed into healthcare improvement practice in ways that are understood to be relevant and useful by professionals and practitioners must, in some sense, be insiders. They must learn to understand and speak the language of improvement, to understand how its practitioners think about what they are doing, and have a sense of the internal dynamics of the field: What are its defining ideas and concepts? What are the central disagreements and tensions at play? What is its history and how has it changed over time?

The starting point for such philosophers, if they wish to be heard, must be observation and understanding of the practice itself. Philosophers might also take on some of the concerns of practitioners – indeed the motivation for their engagement with a field such as improvement might well be to contribute to the aims and practices of healthcare improvement. We have been describing philosophy as a critical (though ideally constructive) force. But if the criticism is not intelligible by practitioners, either because it misunderstands or misrepresents practice, or because it addresses issues which they do not consider relevant, then it is not clear that such philosophical work is meaningfully engaged. To engage effectively in healthcare improvement, philosophers need to do so as relative insiders so they can be adequately responsive to goals and activities internal to improvement practice.

The value of philosophers being insiders is not only to persuade others of their relevance, but also to secure the actual relevance of their conceptual and ethical arguments. While some ethical theorizing uses hypothetical thought experiments and abstracts away from real-world complexity, applied ethicists and especially bioethicists have long emphasized the need for their work to start from observation and understanding of the behaviours, codes, conventions and roles that are internal to the social practices and systems that they are studying. As bioethicist Arthur Caplan stresses: 'It is simply naive to think that a well-trained philosopher can step boldly into the emergency room or neonatal unit and immediately dissolve moral conundrums by dint of expertise in moral theory.'[22] This reflects the idea that any analysis of how people *should* behave must take as its starting point what they already do and think. This doesn't necessarily imply a radically anti-theoretical metaethics: moral theories, including mid-level and high-level principles, may well be a valuable part of philosophical analysis of social activities, but it does suggest that philosophers should continue to look to practise as a basis and sounding board for their theoretical work. Jonathan Wolff calls this approach 'engaged philosophy', emphasizing the value of 'starting from here' rather than beginning with an idealized and unrealistic picture of the world.[23] However, this is not to undermine the value of longer-term projects which aim to shift and shape the values that are endorsed and promoted by practitioners – indeed, as discussed in Chapter 8, this might be some of the most important work that applied philosophers can do. But it cannot take place without close engagement with the reality of the here and now, including the attitudes and beliefs of practitioners.

However, philosophers are not merely insiders; they sit outside of improvement practice in a number of ways. Perhaps most obviously, they are typically employed by institutions such as universities which are not specifically engaged in healthcare improvement. Healthcare improvement is unlikely to be part of their job description, or the job description of their managers, and they are not institutionally incentivized to participate in improvement activities. They thus have less personal investment in the specific methods, approaches and norms of improvement as a field of practice. This distance allows philosophers a critical freedom to question norms of practice that may be less accessible for those working within healthcare or healthcare improvement institutions. It might be more difficult for improvers to engage in such critique not only when their acculturation to improvement norms makes it harder for them to discern the assumptions that are being made, but also when criticism is implicitly or explicitly quashed by strong institutional incentives to participate in improvement activities.

Philosophers also sit outside of improvement practice in less literal ways. While improvement practitioners will be expected if not required to use a professionally approved set of methods and approaches to conduct their work, philosophers come to the table with a different set of disciplinary expectations, which allow them to ask a different and broader range of questions. Philosophers who have not been trained in improvement techniques and approaches will likely come to improvement with a more expansive notion of 'good' and 'better' healthcare than is typically accommodated in improvement activities, connecting healthcare improvement to a wide range of social and ethical issues. They may be better able to notice and look beyond institutional boundaries and highlight the implications of improvement activities in 'non-health-related' social spheres. Philosophers engaging with improvement practice need not adopt the goals of practitioners – though they should be attentive to them – but rather can engage in critical reflection on them with a view to constructive change and even transformation of the field. Many of the difficult and subversive philosophical questions that can be asked of practitioners will interrogate and challenge currently prevailing aims and forms of improvement practice.

This 'insider-outsider' stance provides a particularly good platform for posing potentially destabilizing questions, because it affords philosophers a different and broader perspective on healthcare and improvement. It is important to highlight that we are not talking about destabilizing activity that seeks to undermine or thwart improvement, but rather which seeks to understand whether its ends might better be served in different ways, or whether there are better ways of conceptualizing its ends. The sceptical, subversive avenues available to philosophers mirror, and can potentially support, the sceptical currents that are already built into healthcare improvement activities. And when improvement activities become institutionalized and are in danger of ossifying or otherwise losing some of their sceptical, critical force, philosophers can offer reminders of the assumptions that characterize the field and alternative ways of seeing things.

9.4 Concluding thoughts

As well as seeking to establish a role – or number of roles – for philosophy and philosophers in healthcare improvement, we have also endeavoured to express and explore some counter-cultural and radical ideas about improvement. Most significantly, we have highlighted the importance of thinking about improvement with a view to the long-term and looking outside of narrowly defined institutional and clinical outcomes when trying to understand healthcare processes. And we have emphasized the ways that improvement is deeply and inevitably characterized by high degrees of interpretability and potential disagreement, making it essential for improvers to exhibit humility and appropriate caution in their claims about what is better and why. While we have undoubtedly emphasized the ambiguity, uncertainty and contestation inherent both in claims made about healthcare improvement and actions taken on the basis of such claims, we see this as having the potential to strengthen improvement practice. The evaluative components of improvement activities exist whether they are recognized and embraced or not. But the normative consciousness we have been calling for means acknowledging and welcoming them, so that improvement practice can be much more sensitive to what is at stake – and whose interests are at stake – in decisions about how to design and operate healthcare systems.

In highlighting the potential ways in which philosophy can improve improvement we definitely do not want to suggest that its chief function is to import concerns that are wholly absent from the field. As we have indicated, many of the concerns we have discussed resonate with existing currents including, for example, valuable work on explanatory complexity and foundation-questioning critical social sciences within improvement scholarship. Philosophy complements these currents by encouraging systematic attention to, and explicit debate around, normativity and the conceptual and ethical bases of improvement. In addition to these theoretical resonances there are significant links between the broad philosophical approach we have taken and many influential elements of improvement practice. These include, for example, practical activities that emphasize the sharing of perspectives between stakeholders, conversational dialogue and relational concerns. Practices of these kinds might reasonably be valued because they add respect, warmth and humanity into the field and because they are instrumentally valuable in helping to oil the wheels of change. But bringing a philosophical lens to bear on them shows how – if carefully considered and enacted – they can also be a crucial means of approaching and achieving rigour, and one which philosophical thinking can strengthen. This is not only because better decisions reflecting multiple factors may be reached but also because it is simply more rigorous to have a clear sense, in the process, of what kinds of quality dimensions and whose interests and perspectives are being foregrounded, or relatively side-lined, and why.

In places, our stance towards improvement as a field of practice might be thought to be overly suspicious or pessimistic. We do, indeed, worry – as have others – that much that is labelled 'improvement' is deeply ambiguous, yielding few or no benefits, or generating high costs, or being poorly coordinated and misaligned with broader system-level efforts to change things for the better. The ways that health systems and their outcomes are characterized for the purposes of improvement can be extremely limited, failing to attend to much of what matters. But this does not reflect a deeper pessimism about improvement *per se*. Rather, we think that any attempts to understand what good healthcare looks like, and how to make it better, must reflect and accommodate the extraordinary complexity of health systems. One implication of this is that there may not be very clear or definitive answers to questions about what is good or better, and decisions about what to do need to take seriously this uncertainty. Moreover, attempts to understand what good healthcare looks like must engage fully with the ethical dimensions of improvement, which should seek not just to serve the purposes of healthcare as reflected in normal practice or defined in official documentation, but to think about the social purposes of healthcare more broadly. Health systems have the potential to support not just health but well-being, equality, trust, solidarity and sustainability, and to demonstrate not just technical competence and value for money, but also care, respect, compassion, wisdom, foresight and resourcefulness. Healthcare systems are human systems and, as such, should be humane systems. We think that efforts to improve them should place this humanity at their centre, even – and perhaps especially – when it exposes the messy, ambiguous and contested terrain with which improvers and improvement activities must contend.

NOTES

Chapter 1

1   We use 'technicist' to refer to a (sometimes undue) emphasis on technical questions that obscures the central importance of value judgements in the field.

2   Mitchell et al. (2023).

3   Gilbert (2020); Loveday (2020).

4   Presentation given by Martin Marshall to 5th Annual Conference of the Society of Acute Medicine, London.

5   Ovretveit et al. (2021); Nilsen et al. (2022).

6   Sackett et al. (1996); Guyatt et al. (2004).

7   Nilsen (2015).

8   Healthcare Quality Improvement Partnership (2015).

9   Horizons NHS (2021).

10   For example: King's Improvement Science (2018); Centre for Effective Services (2022); University of Washington (2023).

11   Illustrative examples, from a vast range of work in political philosophy, include: Plato (1974); Young (1990); Rawls (1999); Sen (2009).

12   Illustrative examples of writing on virtues and ethics include: Aristotle [1998]; Hursthouse (1991); Oakley and Cocking (2001); Shafer-Landau (2007).

13   MacIntyre (2007).

14   However, we note that many people in the healthcare improvement field use the term 'science' to encompass an eclectic mixture of forms of expertise and largely to indicate the importance of concerns such as systematicity or auditability – values that are central not only in science but also in other forms of inquiry and public action.

15   In this chapter we continue as if the distinction between facts and values is a relatively clear and clean one. But it is not, and certainly not in relation

to the themes we are discussing. A descriptive account of 'the facts' of healthcare will be a description of human institutions and activities which embody purposes and values and which can only be described in language that has evaluative dimensions. We will explore the intersection further in Chapter 2. For further consideration of the interconnectedness of facts and values, see for example Putnam (2002); Sayer (2011).

16   Institute of Medicine (2001) p1.

17   Institute of Medicine (2001) p2.

18   Institute of Medicine (2001) p25.

19   Institute of Medicine (2001) p28.

20   Institute of Medicine (2001) pp5–6.

21   Dixon-Woods (2019) p1.

22   Dixon-Woods (2019) p1.

23   Fraser (2007).

24   Scaccia and Scott (2021); Sun et al. (2014).

25   Allen et al. (2016).

26   'Technical paradigm' is used here more as an 'ideal type' rather than a 'real-world' category. In practice, outlooks and approaches are often hybrid.

27   Dixon-Woods and Martin (2016).

28   Lawton and Thomas (2022).

Chapter 2

1   Gillespie et al. (2023).

2   The authors of the SDOH screening study cite evidence that doctors can work effectively on social determinants in the kind of ways they are proposing, whilst also suggesting that more, and more rigorous, research needs to be done in this area. There is no shortage of exemplars. In UK primary care, for example, the close involvement of doctors in joint working with, and referring to, diverse agencies supporting social needs was exemplified from the mid-1980s by the work of The Bromley by Bow Centre.

3   There is a very substantial body of literature and debate in this area which, for the most part, we do not address in this book. For current purposes we simply note that characterizing the social world is not straightforward and that researchers arguing for the rigour of their approach need to acknowledge that there are competing conceptions of rigour.

4   Braithwaite et al. (2017).

5   Meadows and Wright (2008).

6   See, for example, UK National Screening Committee (2022); Wilson and Jungner (1968).

7   Gillespie et al. (2023) p10.

8   Gillespie et al. (2023) p2.

9   Plant et al. (2009).

10   Garg et al. (2023).

11   Go (2023).

12   Carter (2018).

13   See, for example, Harvey et al. (2011).

Chapter 3

1   Agency for Healthcare Research and Quality (2022); Australian Commission on Safety and Quality in Health Care (2023); Care Quality Commission (2023).

2   World Health Organization (2018).

3   Institute of Medicine (1990) p4; Council of Europe (1997).

4   Cribb et al. (2020).

5   Shewhart (1925).

6   Now more commonly referred to as PDSA (Plan–Do–Study–Act), as described in Chapter 1. Deming (1986).

7   Power (1999).

8   Maxwell (1984).

9   Institute of Medicine (2001).

10   Cartwright and Runhardt (2014).

11   Institute of Medicine (2001); National Quality Board (2021); World Health Organization (2018).

12   Roberts (2013).

13   Donabedian (1966) p167.

14   Institute of Medicine (2001); World Health Organization (2018); National Quality Board (2021).

15 Care Quality Commission (2022).

16 UK Government (2012).

17 Care Quality Commission (2013).

18 National Quality Board (2016).

19 Sen (1987).

20 Institute of Medicine (2001) p5.

21 National Quality Board (2016) p2.

22 Hollnagel et al. (2015).

23 Star and Griesemer (1989).

Chapter 4

1 As indicated in Chapter 3, the framing of good healthcare in terms of 'quality' itself reflects a normative stance. For now, we set aside the question of whether and when we should use a quality framing at all and assume that we are broadly thinking of healthcare improvement as a matter of improving quality. Towards the end of this chapter, however, we will suggest some limitations to this approach.

2 Latour (1986).

3 Net Domestic Product is calculated by subtracting the estimated cost of depletion and wear-and-tear of capital stock like buildings, equipment and supplies from GDP.

4 We thank Sonya Crowe and Martyn Utley for very helpful discussions about efficiency in the context of home healthcare. See also Mitchell et al. (2024).

5 Alexander (2009).

6 Institute of Medicine (2001) p40.

7 Alexander (2009).

8 Jonsen (1978).

9 Kuzel et al. (2004); Sokol-Hessner et al. (2015).

10 Kuzel et al. (2004).

11 Sokol-Hessner et al. (2015).

12 Simpson (2013).

13 Feinberg (1990).

14 We stress that whether or not some more minor dignitary harms including, for example, particular instances of disrespect, count as harmful in a patient safety-relevant sense, they always have relevance to assessing care quality because of their significance for person-centredness and equality. See Entwistle et al. (2024).

15 Hansson (2013).

16 Mill [1859] (1974).

17 Pettit (2014).

18 Halligan and Zecevic (2011).

Chapter 5

1 Braveman and Gruskin (2003); Young (2001).

2 Gerteis et al. (1993); Mead and Bower (2000); Stewart et al. (2013).

3 Leplege et al. (2007).

4 Byrne et al. (2020); McCormack and McCance (2006).

5 Brooker (2003); Dewing (2002).

6 Little et al. (2001).

7 Freeth (2007); Mezzich (2006).

8 Gerteis et al. (1993); Leplege et al. (2007); Mead and Bower (2000); Stewart et al. (2013).

9 Entwistle et al. (2001); Kahneman (2003); Kahneman and Thaler (2006).

10 Entwistle et al. (2001); Rice and Shorey-Fennell (2020).

11 Braveman and Gruskin (2003) p254.

12 Pelzang (2010) p912.

13 Wittgenstein (1986).

14 Gallie (1955).

15 Pflueger (2015).

16 Medina (2013); Potter (2022).

17 Pflueger (2015).

Chapter 6

1   Wilegoda et al. (2016).

2   Schulpen and Lombarts (2007).

3   This is similar to SDOH screening study discussed in Chapter 2. See also Singh and Zhu (2020).

4   See, for example, the 'WHAM' project: https://www.whamproject.co.uk (accessed 5 June 2005).

5   We imagine virtually no-one outside of academic circles 'does ethics' by conscious reference to ethical theory and, we suggest, there are grounds for being sceptical about the wisdom of anyone who relies heavily on theoretical abstractions. Nonetheless, the ethical theories mentioned here identify important ethical ideas and values which do commonly feature in decision-making and justifications for action. We say more about the limits of ethical theory and theorizing in Chapter 7.

6   Holohan (2019).

7   Singh and Cribb (2021).

8   Lawton and Thomas (2022); Thomas (2020).

9   This point draws on a Q Community Philosophy and Ethics Special Interest Group discussion event held on 7 June 2023.

10   Mitchell et al. (2021b).

11   Wilfond and Ravitsky (2005).

12   This idea is often attributed to Don Berwick of the Institute for Healthcare Improvement, but Berwick himself has said the original source was a nurse pithily summing up an IHI course he was leading.

13   Wilson and Hunter (2010).

14   Jennings (2007).

15   Msuya (2003).

16   Liberati et al. (2019).

17   Dixon-Woods and Pronovost (2016).

18   https://www.cqc.org.uk/about-us/how-we-do-our-job/ratings (accessed 5 June 2025).

19   For example, Pålsson (2020).

20   Sholl et al. (2019); Hodkinson et al. (2007).

21   Wolff (2019).

22 See Sinclair (2022).

23 Jecker (2013); Sheehan (2007).

24 Mitchell et al. (2021a).

Chapter 7

1 Emanuel and Emanuel (1996).

2 Weale (2011) p76.

3 Bovens (2007); Schedler (1999).

4 Lynn et al. (2007).

5 The focus here is on accountability within institutions, where there are usually recognized reporting hierarchies. This says little about how to think about accountability for cross-institutional or system-wide improvement activities.

6 Lynn et al. (2007) p680.

7 Lynn et al. (2007) Table 1.

8 Lynn et al. (2007) p666.

9 Lynn et al. (2007) Table 2.

10 For example, Fiscella et al. (2015).

11 Lynn et al. (2007) p668.

12 Lynn et al. (2007) p669.

13 See Table 3 of Lynn et al. (2007).

14 Lynn et al. (2007) p672.

15 See, for example, Oakley and Cocking (2001).

16 MacIntyre (2007).

17 Oakley and Cocking (2001); Pellegrino (1995).

18 Lucas and Nacer (2015).

19 Lucas and Nacer (2015) p12.

20 Lucas and Nacer (2015) p8.

21 Dixon-Woods (2014).

22 Hursthouse (2006).

23 https://www.ihi.org/resources/how-improve-model-improvement (accessed 5 May 2025).

24 Pflueger (2015).

25 Snow [1959] (2012).

26 Cribb and Woodcock (2022).

27 Oakeshott (1962) p197.

28 See Martin et al. (2018) on 'soft intelligence'.

29 Sliwa (2023).

30 Francis (2013).

31 Vincent et al. (2014).

32 Goldman et al. (2023).

33 Goldman et al. (2023) p475.

34 Cribb et al. (2022).

35 Nussbaum (1990); Kerasidou et al. (2021).

36 Cribb et al. (2023).

Chapter 8

1 Delivery and revisionary perspectives may be difficult to disentangle in practice because, for example, for a change to be able to 'spread' it will likely have to go deeper than surface behaviour change.

2 Seedhouse (1986).

3 Nordenfelt (1987).

4 In the UK health visitors are specialist nurses or midwives, with additional community public health training, who work with pregnant people, young infants and parents.

5 Boorse (1977); Hausman (2012, 2014). Of course even if one accepts that health can and should be defined non-normatively it is still possible to conclude that healthcare practice is itself normatively constituted – the position we have taken throughout – because (a) there is no reason to assume that the only purpose of healthcare is to advance health in this non-normative sense and (b) healthcare actors operate in social fields and work with and for people who value things and cannot neatly separate their work from these normative contexts and considerations.

6 Venkatapuram (2011).

7   In the full account the capability to be healthy is characterized as a second-order or 'meta-capability', in other words the capability to exercise other key capabilities, which Venkatapuram specifies using Martha Nussbaum's (2011) list of 'central human capabilities'. The central human capabilities involve people having both the internal and external resources needed for opportunities to, for example, reason about their life, express themselves and their emotions, form ties with people, hold property, participate in political processes and play, etc.

8   Valles (2018).

9   Seedhouse (1986), cover text.

10 Carel (2016).

11 See, for example, the Health Foundation (2024).

12 See, for example, Engman (2019).

13 Institute for Healthcare Improvement (2024); Bridges et al. (2017); Devi et al. (2023).

14 Rogers (2020).

15 Fornell (2022).

16 American Medical Association (2022).

17 Royal College of Physicians (2023).

18 Franz et al. (2019).

19 Bajaj et al. (2023).

20 Thomas and Cosford (2010).

21 Centre for Sustainable Healthcare (2024).

22 Nielsen et al. (2021).

23 Bajaj et al. (2023).

24 Thiele (2024).

25 Thiele (2024) p5.

26 Thiele (2024) p3.

27 Thiele (2024) p9.

28 As in Institute of Medicine (2001).

29 Nuriddin et al. (2020).

30 Nuriddin et al. (2020) p950.

31 NHS Confederation (2022a).

32 Rondini et al. (2021).

33 Onwuegbuzia (2024).

34 Rondini et al. (2021) p67.

35 Knight et al. (2023).

36 Connor and Dhaliwal (2023) p1.

37 Connor and Dhaliwal (2023) p1.

38 We stress that some 'trade-offs' may be needed in prioritizing quality approaches, but that is a different matter. In the case of 'trade-offs', tensions are being recognized and consciously, if imperfectly, managed.

39 Ray and Davis (2021).

40 Ricks et al. (2022) p1990.

41 Hassen et al. (2021) p1/15.

42 Hassen et al. (2021) p12/15.

43 Paine et al. (2021) p1/17.

44 Jones et al. (2019a).

45 Jones et al. (2019b).

46 Jones et al. (2019b).

47 The Health Foundation (n.d.).

48 Jones and Pereira (2023).

49 Hardie et al. (2022).

50 Papoutsi et al. (2024).

51 Papoutsi et al. (2024) p4.

52 Papoutsi et al. (2024) p5.

Chapter 9

1 Mitchell et al. (2023).

2 Carter (2018) p190.

3 Wolff (2019); Mitchell et al. (2021a).

4 Mitchell et al. (2019).

5 Braithwaite et al. (2017).

6 Midgley (1992) p139.

7 Midgley (1992) p139.

8 Midgley (1992) p139.

9 Hollnagel et al. (2015).

10 The Royal College of Surgeons of England (n.d.).

11 Chou et al. (2015).

12 Beauchamp and Childress (2019).

13 Arras (2009); Jonsen (1991).

14 Midgley (1992) p141.

15 Wolff (2019).

16 Hyde (1998).

17 Hyde (1998) p7.

18 Lock (2002).

19 Lock (2002).

20 Lock (2002).

21 Mitchell et al. (2023).

22 Caplan (1980) p27.

23 Wolff (2019).

REFERENCES

Agency for Healthcare Research and Quality (2022). Agency for Healthcare Research and Quality: A profile. https://www.ahrq.gov/cpi/about/profile/index.html (accessed 23 November 2023).

Alexander, J.K. (2009). The concept of efficiency: An historical analysis. In: Meijers, A. (Ed.), *Philosophy of technology and engineering sciences*. Amsterdam: Elsevier, pp. 1007–30.

Allen, D., Braithwaite, J., Sandall, J., Waring, J. (Eds.) (2016). *The sociology of healthcare safety and quality*. Oxford: Wiley-Blackwell.

American Medical Association (2022). AMA strengthens commitment to combatting climate crisis. Press Release, 15 November 2022. https://www.ama-assn.org/press-center/ama-press-releases/ama-strengthens-commitment-combatting-climate-crisis (accessed 13 June 2025).

Aristotle [1925] (1998). *The Nicomachean ethics*. Oxford: Oxford University Press.

Arras, J.D. (2009). A case approach. In: Kuhse, H. and Singer, P. (Eds.), *A companion to bioethics*. Malden, MA: Wiley, pp. 117–25.

Australian Commission on Safety and Quality in Health Care (2023). *The NSQHS standards*. https://www.safetyandquality.gov.au/standards/nsqhs-standards (accessed 23 November 2023).

Bajaj, K., Musser, L., Wei, E., Bailey, J., Jones, A., Vinoya-Chung, C. (2023). Integrating environmental sustainability into the quality and safety agenda: Early lessons learned. Institute for Healthcare Improvement Blog. https://www.ihi.org/insights/integrating-environmental-sustainability-quality-and-safety-agenda-early-lessons-learned (accessed 30 April 2024).

Beauchamp, T.L., Childress, J.F. (2019). *Principles of biomedical ethics*, 8th edn. New York, NY: Oxford University Press.

Boorse, C. (1977). Health as a theoretical concept. *Philosophy of Science*, 44:542–73. https://www.jstor.org/stable/186939

Bovens, M. (2007). Analysing and assessing accountability: A conceptual framework. *European Law Journal*, 13:447–68. https://doi.org/10.1111/j.1468-0386.2007.00378.x

Braithwaite, J., Churruca, K., Ellis, L.A., Long, J., Clay-Williams, R., Damen, N., Herkes, J., Pomare, C., Ludlow, K. (2017). *Complexity science in healthcare — aspirations, approaches, applications and accomplishments: A white paper*. Sydney: Australian Institute of Health Innovation, Macquarie University.

Braveman, P., Gruskin, S. (2003). Defining equity in health. *Journal of Epidemiology and Community Health*, 57:254–8. https://doi.org/10.1136/jech.57.4.254

Bridges, J., May, C., Fuller, A., Griffiths, P., Wigley, W., Gould, L., Barker, H., Libberton, P. (2017). Optimising impact and sustainability: A qualitative process evaluation of a complex intervention targeted at compassionate care. *BMJ Quality & Safety*, 26:970–7. https://doi.org/10.1136/bmjqs-2017-006702

Brooker, D. (2003). What is person-centred care in dementia? *Reviews in Clinical Gerontology*, 13:215–22. https://doi.org/10.1017/S095925980400108X

Byrne, A.-L., Baldwin, A., Harvey, C. (2020). Whose centre is it anyway? Defining person-centred care in nursing: An integrative review. *PLOS ONE*, 15:e0229923. https://doi.org/10.1371/journal.pone.0229923

Caplan, A.L. (1980). Ethical engineers need not apply: The state of applied ethics today. *Science, Technology and Human Values*, 5(4):24–32. https://doi.org/10.1177/016224398000500403

Care Quality Commission (2013). *A new start: Consultation on changes to the way CQC regulates, inspects and monitors care.* London: Care Quality Commission.

Care Quality Commission (2022). *The five key questions we ask.* https://www.cqc.org.uk/what-we-do/how-we-do-our-job/five-key-questions-we-ask (accessed 28 July 2022).

Care Quality Commission (2023). *CQC: About us.* https://www.cqc.org.uk/about-us (accessed 23 November 2023).

Carel, H. (2016). *Phenomenology of illness.* Oxford: Oxford University Press.

Carter, S.M. (2018). Valuing healthcare improvement: Implicit norms, explicit normativity, and human agency. *Health Care Analysis*, 26(2):189–205. https://doi.org/10.1007/s10728-017-0350-x

Cartwright, N., Runhardt, R. (2014). Measurement. In: Cartwright, N. and Montuschi, E. (Eds.), *Philosophy of social science: A new introduction.* Oxford: Oxford University Press, pp. 265–87.

Centre for Effective Services (2022). *Implementation frameworks provide a conceptual model of implementation.* https://implementation.effectiveservices.org/frameworks (accessed 23 November 2023).

Centre for Sustainable Healthcare (2024). Sustainability in Quality Improvement (SusQI). https://sustainablehealthcare.org.uk/susqi (accessed 30 April 2024).

Chou, E., Abboudi, H., Shamim Khan, M., Dasgupta, P., Ahmed, K. (2015). Should surgical outcomes be published? *Journal of the Royal Society of Medicine*, 108(4):127–35. https://doi.org/10.1177/0141076815578652

Connor, D.M., Dhaliwal, G. (2023). Moving upstream to address diagnostic disparities. *BMJ Quality & Safety*, 32(11):620–2. https://doi.org/10.1136/bmjqs-2023-016130

Council of Europe (1997). *The development and implementation of quality improvement systems (QIS) in health care. Recommendation No. R (97) 17 and explanatory memorandum.* Strasbourg: Council of Europe.

Cribb, A., Woodcock, T. (2022). Measuring with quality: The example of person-centred care. *Journal of Health Services Research and Policy*, 27(2):151–6. https://doi.org/10.1177/13558196211054278

Cribb, A., Entwistle, V., Mitchell, P. (2020). What does 'quality' add? Towards an ethics of healthcare improvement. *Journal of Medical Ethics*, 46(2):118–22. https://doi.org/10.1136/medethics-2019-105635

Cribb, A., Entwistle, V., Mitchell, P. (2022). Talking it better: Conversations and normative complexity in healthcare improvement. *Medical Humanities*, 48(1):85–93. https://doi.org/10.1136/medhum-2020-012129

Cribb, A., Entwistle, V., Mitchell, P. (2023). Varieties of improvement expertise: Knowledge and contestation in health-care improvement. *Sociology of Health and Illness*, 45(4):734–53. https://doi.org/10.1111/1467-9566.13616

Crisp, R., Slote, M.A. (Eds.) (1997). *Virtue ethics.* Oxford: Oxford University Press.

Deming, E. (1986). *Out of the crisis.* Cambridge, MA: Massachusetts Institute of Technology.

Devi, R., Martin, G.P., Banerjee, J., Gladman, J.R.F., Dening, T., Barat, A., Gordon, A.L. (2023). Sustaining interventions in care homes initiated by quality improvement projects: A qualitative study. *BMJ Quality & Safety*, 32(11):665–75. https://doi.org/10.1136/bmjqs-2021-014345

Dewing, J. (2002). From ritual to relationship: A person-centred approach to consent in qualitative research with older people who have a dementia. *Dementia*, 1:157–71. https://doi.org/10.1177/147130120200100204

Dixon-Woods, M. (2014). *The problem of context in quality improvement.* London: Health Foundation, London, UK. https://www.health.org.uk/sites/default/files/PerspectivesOnContextDixonWoodsTheProblemOfContextInQuality Improvement.pdf (accessed 24 June 2025).

Dixon-Woods, M. (2019). How to improve healthcare improvement: An essay by Mary Dixon-Woods. *BMJ*, 367:I5514. https://doi.org/10.1136/bmj.I5514

Dixon-Woods, M., Martin, G.P. (2016). Does quality improvement improve quality? *Future Hospital Journal*, 3(3):191–4. https://doi.org/10.7861/futurehosp.3-3-191

Dixon-Woods, M., Pronovost, P.J. (2016). Patient safety and the problem of many hands. *BMJ Quality & Safety*, 25(7):485–8. https://doi.org/10.1136/bmjqs-2016-005232

Donabedian, A. (1966). Evaluating the quality of medical care. *Milbank Memorial Fund Quarterly*, 44(3):166–206. https://doi.org/10.2307/3348969

Emanuel, E.J., Emanuel, L.L. (1996). What is accountability in health care? *Annals of Internal Medicine*, 124(2):229–39. https://doi.org/10.7326/0003-4819-124-2-199601150-00007

Engman, A. (2019). Embodiment and the foundation of biographical disruption. *Social Science and Medicine*, 225:120–7. https://doi.org/10.1016/j.socscimed.2019.02.019

Entwistle, V., Cribb, A., Mitchell, P. (2024). Tackling disrespect in healthcare: The relevance of socio-relational equality. *Journal of Health Services Research and Policy*, 29(1):42–50. https://doi.org.10.1177/13558196231187961

Entwistle, V., Skea, Z., O'Donnell, M. (2001). Decisions about treatment: Interpretations of two measures of control by women having a hysterectomy. *Social Science and Medicine*, 53(6):721–32. https://doi.org/10.1016/S0277-9536(00)00382-8

Feinberg, J. (1990). *Harm to others: The moral limits of the criminal law*. New York, NY: Oxford University Press.

Fiscella, K., Tobin, J.N., Carroll, J.K., He, H., Ogedegbe, G. (2015). Ethical oversight in quality improvement and quality improvement research: New approaches to promote a learning health care system. *BMC Medical Ethics*, 16:63. https://doi.org/10.1186/s12910-015-0056-2

Fornell, D. (2022). AMA declares climate change a public health crisis. *HealthExec*, 16 June 2022. https://healthexec.com/topics/healthcare-management/healthcare-policy/ama-declares-climate-change-public-health-crisis (accessed 24 June 2025).

Francis, R. (2013). *Report of the Mid Staffordshire NHS Foundation Trust Public Inquiry – Volume 3: Present and Future*. London: The Stationery Office.

Franz, B., Skinner, D., Wynn, J., Kelleher, K. (2019). Urban hospitals as anchor institutions: Frameworks for medical sociology. *Socius: Sociological Research for a Dynamic World*, 5. https://doi.org/10.1177/2378023118817981

Fraser, N. (2007). Reframing justice in a globalizing world. In: Held, D. and Kaya, A. (Eds.), *Global inequality: Patterns and explanations*. Cambridge: Polity Press, pp. 252–72.

Freeth, R. (2007). *Humanising psychiatry and mental health care: The challenge of the person-centred approach*. Oxford: Radcliffe Publishing.

Gallie, W.B. (1955). Essentially contested concepts. *Proceedings of the Aristotelian Society*, 56:167–98. https://www.jstor.org/stable/4544562

Garg, A., LeBlanc, A., Raphael, J.L. (2023). Inadequacy of current screening measures for health-related social needs. *JAMA*, 330(10):915–16. https://doi.org/10.1001/jama.2023.13948

Gerteis, M., Edgman-Levitan, S., Daley, J., Delbanco, T.L. (1993). *Through the patient's eyes: Theoretical development of what defines quality from the patients' perspective*. San Francisco, CA: Jossey-Bass.

Gilbert, H.A. (2020). Florence Nightingale's Environmental Theory and its influence on contemporary infection control. *Collegian*, 27(6):626–33. https://doi.org/10.1016/j.colegn.2020.09.006

Gillespie, C., Wilhite, J.A., Hanley, K., Hardowar, K., Altshuler, L., Fisher, H., Porter, B., Wallach, A., Zabar, S. (2023). Addressing social determinants of health in primary care: A quasi-experimental study using unannounced standardised patients to evaluate the impact of audit/feedback on physicians' rates of identifying and responding to social needs. *BMJ Quality & Safety*, 32(11):632–43. https://doi.org/10.1136/bmjqs-2021-013904

Go, J. (2023). The expressive function of healthcare. *Journal of Ethics*, 27:329–53. https://doi.org/10.1007/s10892-023-09433-w

Goldman, J., Rotteau, L., Flintoft, V., Jeffs, L., Baker, G.R. (2023). Measurement and monitoring of safety framework: A qualitative study of implementation through a Canadian learning collaborative. *BMJ Quality & Safety*, 32(8): 470–8. https://doi.org/10.1136/bmjqs-2022-015017

Guyatt, G., Cook, D., Haynes, B. (2004). Evidence based medicine has come a long way. *BMJ*, 329:990–1. https://doi.org/10.1136/bmj.329.7473.990

Halligan, M., Zecevic, A. (2011). Safety culture in healthcare: A review of concepts, dimensions, measures and progress. *BMJ Quality & Safety*, 20(4):338–43. https://doi.org/10.1136/bmjqs.2010.040964

Hansson, S.O. (2013). *The ethics of risk: Ethical analysis in an uncertain world.* Basingstoke: Springer.

Hardie, T., Horton, T., Thornton, N., Home, J., Pereira, P. (2022). *Developing learning health systems in the UK: Priorities for action.* London: The Health Foundation. https://www.health.org.uk/reports-and-analysis/reports/developing-learning-health-systems-in-the-uk-priorities-for-action.

Harvey, G., Fitzgerald, L., Fielden, S., McBride, A., Waterman, H., Bamford, D., Kislov, R., Boaden, R. (2011). The NIHR collaboration for leadership in applied health research and care (CLAHRC) for Greater Manchester: Combining empirical, theoretical and experiential evidence to design and evaluate a large-scale implementation strategy. *Implementation Science*, 6:96. https://doi.org/10.1186/1748-5908-6-96

Hassen, N., Lofters, A., Michael, S., Mall, A., Pinto, A.D., Rackal, J. (2021). Implementing anti-racism interventions in healthcare settings: A scoping review. *International Journal of Environmental Research and Public. Health*, 18:2993. https://doi.org/10.3390/ijerph18062993

Hausman, D.M. (2012). Health, naturalism, and functional efficiency. *Philosophy of Science*, 79(4):519–41. https://doi.org/10.1086/668005

Hausman, D.M. (2014). Health and functional efficiency. *Journal of Medicine and Philosophy*, 39:634–47. https://doi.org/10.1093/jmp/jhu036

Healthcare Quality Improvement Partnership (2015). *A guide to quality improvement methods.* London: HQIP. https://www.hqip.org.uk/wp-content/uploads/2018/02/guide-to-quality-improvement-methods.pdf (accessed 4 April 2025).

Hodkinson, P., Biesta, G., James, D. (2007). Understanding learning cultures. *Educational Review*, 59(4):415–27. https://doi.org/10.1080/00131910701619316

Hollnagel, E., Wears, R.L., Braithwaite, J. (2015). *From Safety-I to Safety-II: A white paper.* University of Southern Denmark, University of Florida, USA, and Macquarie University, Australia. https://www.mq.edu.au/__data/assets/pdf_file/0011/84296/From_Safety_I_to_Safety_II_A_White_Paper.pdf (accessed 26 May 2025).

Holohan, E. (2019). P193 Quality improvement in nursing clinical handover. *Archives of Disease in Childhood*, 104(S3):A235. https://doi.org/10.1136/archdischild-2019-epa.548

Horizons NHS (2021). *Welcome to the Improvement Method Olympics!* http://
horizonsnhs.com/improvementmethodolympics/ (accessed 22 November 2023).

Hursthouse, R. (1991). Virtue theory and abortion. *Philosophy and Public
Affairs*, 20(3):223–46.

Hursthouse, R. (2006). XI – Practical wisdom: A mundane account. *Proceedings
of the Aristotelian Society*, 106(1):285–309. https://doi.org/10.1111/j.1467-
9264.2006.00149.x

Hyde, L. (1998). *Trickster makes this world: Mischief, myth, and art*. New York:
Farrar, Straus and Giroux.

Institute for Healthcare Improvement (2024). *Sustainability Planning Worksheet*.
https://www.ihi.org/resources/tools/sustainability-planning-worksheet
(accessed 30 April 2024).

Institute of Medicine (1990). *Medicare: A strategy for quality assurance, Volume
I*. Washington, DC: National Academies Press. https://doi.org/10.17226/1547

Institute of Medicine (2001). *Crossing the quality chasm: A new health system
for the 21st century*. Washington, DC: National Academy Press. https://doi.
org/10.17226/10027

Jecker, N.S. (2013). The problem with rescue medicine. *Journal of Medicine and
Philosophy*, 38(1):64–81. https://doi.org/10.1093/jmp/jhs056

Jennings, B. (2007). *Health care quality improvement: Ethical and regulatory issues*.
Garrison, NY: Hastings Center. https://www.thehastingscenter.org/wp-content/
uploads/Health-Care-Quality-Improvement.pdf (accessed 27 May 2025).

Jones, B., Pereira, P. (2023). *Improvement as mainstream business: The strategic
case*. London: The Health Foundation.

Jones, L., Fraser, A., Stewart, E. (2019a). Exploring the neglected and hidden
dimensions of large-scale healthcare change. *Sociology of Health and Illness*,
41(7):1221–35. https://doi.org/10.1111/1467-9566.12923

Jones, L., Fraser, A., Stewart, E. (2019b). Why social science can help us to better
understand organisational change in healthcare. *LSE Blog*. URL https://blogs.
lse.ac.uk/impactofsocialsciences/2019/07/08/why-social-science-can-help-
us-to-better-understand-organisational-change-in-healthcare/ (accessed 30
April 2024).

Jonsen, A.R. (1978). Do no harm. *Annals of Internal Medicine*, 88(6):827.
https://doi.org/10.7326/0003-4819-88-6-827

Jonsen, A.R. (1991). Casuistry as methodology in clinical ethics. *Theoretical
Medicine*, 12:295–307. https://doi.org/10.1007/BF00489890

Kahneman, D. (2003). A perspective on judgment and choice: Mapping
bounded rationality. *American Psychologist*, 58(9):697–720. https://doi.
org/10.1037/0003-066X.58.9.697

Kahneman, D., Thaler, R.H. (2006). Anomalies: Utility maximization and
experienced utility. *Journal of Economic Perspectives*, 20(1):221–34. https://
doi.org/10.1257/089533006776526076

Kerasidou, A., Bærøe, K., Berger, Z., Caruso Brown, A.E. (2021). The need for
empathetic healthcare systems. *Journal of Medical Ethics*, 47(12):e27. https://
doi.org/10.1136/medethics-2019-105921

King's Improvement Science (2018). *Implementation science research development (ImpRes) tool: A tool to improve the quality of implementation projects.* London: King's Improvement Science. https://kingsimprovementscience.org/cms-data/resources/ImpRes_guide_December%202018.pdf (accessed 27 May 2025).

Knight, M., Bunch, K., Felker, A., Patel, R., Kotnis, R., Kenyon, S., Kurinczuk, J.J. (2023). *Saving lives, improving mothers' care core report: Lessons learned to inform maternity care from the UK and Ireland confidential enquiries into maternal deaths and morbidity, 2019–2021.* MBRRACE-UK. https://www.npeu.ox.ac.uk/assets/downloads/mbrrace-uk/reports/maternal-report-2023/MBRRACE-UK_Maternal_Compiled_Report_2023.pdf (accessed 25 June 2025).

Kuzel, A.J., Woolf, S.H., Gilchrist, V.J., Engel, J.D., LaVeist, T.A., Vincent, C., Frankel, R.M. (2004). Patient reports of preventable problems and harms in primary health care. *Annals of Family Medicine*, 2(4):333–40. https://doi.org/10.1370/afm.220

Latour, B. (1986). Visualisation and cognition: Drawing things together. In: Long, E. and Kuklick, H. (Eds.), *Knowledge and society: Studies in the sociology of culture past and present (Volume 6).* Greenwich, CT: JAI Press, pp. 1–40.

Lawton, R., Thomas, E.J. (2022). Overcoming the 'self-limiting' nature of QI: Can we improve the quality of patient care while caring for staff? *BMJ Quality & Safety*, 31(12):857–9. https://doi.org/10.1136/bmjqs-2022-015272

Leplege, A., Gzil, F., Cammelli, M., Lefeve, C., Pachoud, B., Ville, I. (2007). Person-centredness: Conceptual and historical perspectives. *Disability and Rehabilitation*, 29(20–21):1555–65. https://doi.org/10.1080/09638280701618661

Liberati, E.G., Tarrant, C., Willars, J., Draycott, T., Winter, C., Chew, S., Dixon-Woods, M. (2019). How to be a very safe maternity unit: An ethnographic study. *Social Science and Medicine*, 223:64–72. https://doi.org/10.1016/j.socscimed.2019.01.035

Little, P., Everitt, H., Williamson, I., Warner, G., Moore, M., Gould, C., Ferrier, K., Payne, S. (2001). Preferences of patients for patient centred approach to consultation in primary care: Observational study. *BMJ*, 322:468. https://doi.org/10.1136/bmj.322.7284.468

Lock, H. (2002). Transformations of the Trickster. *Southern Cross Review*, 18:1–8. https://southerncrossreview.org/18/trickster.htm

Loveday, H.P. (2020). Revisiting Florence Nightingale: International Year of the Nurse and Midwife 2020. *Journal of Infection and Prevention*, 21(1):4–6. https://doi.org/10.1177/1757177419896246

Lucas, B., Nacer, H. (2015). *The habits of an improver. Thinking about learning for improvement in health care.* London: Health Foundation. https://www.health.org.uk/reports-and-analysis/reports/the-habits-of-an-improver (accessed 27 May 2025).

Lynn, J., Baily, M.A., Bottrell, M., Jennings, B., Levine, R.J., Davidoff, F. Casarett, D., Corrigan, J., Fox, E., Wynia, M.K., Agich, G.J., O'Kane, M., Speroff, T., Schyve, P., Batalden, P., Tunis, S., Berlinger, N., Cronenwett, L.,

Fitzmaurice, M., Nevelkoff-Dubler, N., James, B. (2007). The ethics of using quality improvement methods in health Care. *Annals of Internal Medicine*, 146(9):666–73. https://doi.org/10.7326/0003-4819-146-9-200705010-00155

MacIntyre, A.C. (2007). *After virtue: A study in moral theory*, 3rd edn. Notre Dame, IN: University of Notre Dame Press.

Martin, G.P., Aveling, E.-L., Campbell, A., Tarrant, C., Pronovost, P.J., Mitchell, I., Dankers, C., Bates, D., Dixon-Woods, M. (2018). Making soft intelligence hard: A multi-site qualitative study of challenges relating to voice about safety concerns. *BMJ Quality & Safety*, 27(9):710–17. https://doi.org/10.1136/bmjqs-2017-007579

Maxwell, R.J. (1984). Quality assessment in health. *BMJ*, 288:1470–2. https://doi.org/10.1136/bmj.288.6428.1470

McCormack, B., McCance, T.V. (2006). Development of a framework for person-centred nursing. *Journal of Advanced Nursing*, 56(5):472–9. https://doi.org/10.1111/j.1365-2648.2006.04042.x

Mead, N., Bower, P. (2000). Patient-centredness: A conceptual framework and review of the empirical literature. *Social Science and Medicine*, 51(7):1087–110. https://doi.org/10.1016/S0277-9536(00)00098-8

Meadows, D.H., Wright, D. (2008). *Thinking in systems: A primer*. White River Junction, VT: Chelsea Green.

Medina, J. (2013). *The epistemology of resistance: Gender and racial oppression, epistemic injustice, and the social imagination*. Oxford: Oxford University Press. https://doi.org/10.1093/acprof:oso/9780199929023.001.0001

Mezzich, J.E. (2006). Institutional consolidation and global impact: Towards a psychiatry for the person. *World Psychiatry*, 5(2):65–6.

Midgley, M. (1992). Philosophical plumbing. *Royal Institute of Philosophy Supplement*, 33:139–51. https://doi.org/10.1017/S1358246100002319

Mill, J.S. [1859] (1974). *On liberty*. London: Penguin Books.

Mitchell, P., Cribb, A., Entwistle, V.A. (2019). Defining what is good: Pluralism and healthcare quality. *Kennedy Institute of Ethics Journal*, 29(4):367–88. https://dx.doi.org/10.1353/ken.2019.0030.

Mitchell, P., Cribb, A., Entwistle, V. (2021a). Made to measure: The ethics of routine measurement for healthcare improvement. *Health Care Analysis*, 29:39–58. https://doi.org/10.1007/s10728-020-00421-x

Mitchell, P., Cribb, A., Entwistle, V., Singh, G. (2021b). Pushing poverty off limits: Quality improvement and the architecture of healthcare values. *BMC Medical Ethics*, 22:91. https://doi.org/10.1186/s12910-021-00655-x

Mitchell, P., Cribb, A., Entwistle, V. (2023). Truth and consequences. *Metaphilosophy*, 54(4):523–38. https://doi.org/10.1111/meta.12644

Mitchell, P., Cribb, A., Entwistle, V., Crowe, S. (2024). Making ends meet: A conceptual and ethical analysis of efficiency. *Kennedy Institute of Ethics Journal*, 34(1):1–26. http://doi.org/10.1353/ken.2024.a943428

Msuya, J. (2003). *Horizontal and vertical delivery of health services: What are the trade offs?* Washington, DC: World Bank. http://documents.worldbank.org/curated/en/914491468761944686

National Quality Board (2016). *Shared commitment to quality from the National Quality Board. National Quality Board*. https://www.england.nhs.uk/wp-content/uploads/2016/12/nqb-shared-commitment-frmwrk.pdf (accessed 27 May 2025).

National Quality Board (2021). *A shared commitment to quality for those working in health and care systems.* https://www.england.nhs.uk/wp-content/uploads/2021/04/nqb-refreshed-shared-commitment-to-quality.pdf (accessed 27 May 2025).

NHS Confederation (2022a). *Shattered hopes: Black and minority ethnic leaders' experiences of breaking the glass ceiling in the NHS.* https://www.nhsconfed.org/system/files/2022-06/Shattered-hopes-BME-leaders-glass-ceiling-NHS.pdf (accessed 27 May 2025).

NHS Confederation (2022b). *Commit, understand, act: Our anti-racism strategy.* https://www.nhsconfed.org/system/files/2022-11/Commit-understand-act-our-racism-strategy-FNL-4.pdf (accessed 27 May 2025).

Nielsen, L., Bush, O., Steinbach, I. (2021). *Case report: Pioneering early mobilisation in a cardiac intensive care (CICU) unit: A Sustainable Healthcare initiative.* Centre for Sustainable Healthcare. https://networks.sustainablehealthcare.org.uk/sites/default/files/resources/Early%20Mobilisation%20Case%20Report.pdf (accessed 27 May 2025).

Nilsen, P. (2015). Making sense of implementation theories, models and frameworks. *Implementation Science*, 10:53. https://doi.org/10.1186/s13012-015-0242-0

Nilsen, P., Thor, J., Bender, M., Leeman, J., Andersson-Gäre, B., Sevdalis, N. (2022). Bridging the silos: A comparative analysis of implementation science and improvement science. *Frontiers in Health Services*, 1:817750. https://doi.org/10.3389/frhs.2021.817750

Nordenfelt, L. (1987). *On the nature of health: An action-theoretic approach. Philosophy and Medicine.* Dordrecht: Springer-Dordrecht. https://doi.org/10.1007/978-94-015-7768-7

Nuriddin, A., Mooney, G., White, A.I.R. (2020). Reckoning with histories of medical racism and violence in the USA. *The Lancet*, 396(10256):949–51. https://doi.org/10.1016/S0140-6736(20)32032-8

Nussbaum, M.C. (1990). *Love's knowledge: Essays on philosophy and literature.* New York, NY: Oxford University Press.

Nussbaum, M.C. (2011). *Creating capabilities: The human development approach.* Cambridge, MA: Harvard University Press. https://doi.org/10.2307/j.ctt2jbt31

Oakeshott, M. (1962). *Rationalism in politics and other essays.* New York, NY: Rowman.

Oakley, J., Cocking, D. (2001). *Virtue ethics and professional roles.* Cambridge: Cambridge University Press. https://doi.org/10.1017/CBO9780511487118

Onwuegbuzia, A.V. (2024). Digital disparities: How artificial intelligence can facilitate anti-black racism in the US healthcare sector. *International Relations and Diplomacy*, 12(1):40–50. https://doi.org/10.17265/2328-2134/2024.01.005

Ovretveit, J., Mittman, B.S., Rubenstein, L.V., Ganz, D.A. (2021). Combining improvement and implementation sciences and practices for the post

COVID-19 era. *Journal of General Internal Medicine*, 36(11):3503–10. https://doi.org/10.1007/s11606-020-06373-1

Paine, L., De La Rocha, P., Eyssallenne, A.P., Andrews, C.A., Loo, L., Jones, C.P., Collins, A.M., Morse, M. (2021). Declaring racism a public health crisis in the United States: Cure, poison, or both? *Frontiers in Public Health*, 9:676784. https://doi.org/10.3389/fpubh.2021.676784

Pålsson, D. (2020). Securing the floor but not raising the ceiling? Operationalising care quality in the inspection of residential care for children in Sweden. *European Journal of Social Work*, 23:118–30. https://doi.org/10.1080/13691457.2018.1476331

Papoutsi, C., Greenhalgh, T., Marjanovic, S. (2024). *Approaches to spread, scale-up, and sustainability*. In series: Cambridge Elements: Improving quality and safety in healthcare. Cambridge: Cambridge University Press. https://doi.org/10.1017/9781009326049

Pellegrino, E.D. (1995). Toward a virtue-based normative ethics for the health professions. *Kennedy Institute of Ethics Journal*, 5:253–77. https://doi.org/10.1353/ken.0.0044

Pelzang, R. (2010). Time to learn: Understanding patient-centred care. *British Journal of Nursing*, 19:912–17. https://doi.org/10.12968/bjon.2010.19.14.49050

Pettit, P. (2014). *Just freedom: A moral compass for a complex world.* New York, NY: W.W. Norton.

Pflueger, D. (2015). Accounting for quality: On the relationship between accounting and quality improvement in healthcare. *BMC Health Services Research*, 15:178. https://doi.org/10.1186/s12913-015-0769-4

Plant, R., Taylor-Gooby, P., Lesser, A. (2009). *Political philosophy and social welfare*. London: Routledge. https://doi.org/10.4324/9780203092262

Plato (1974). *The Republic*, 2nd edn. London: Penguin.

Potter, N.N. (2022). The virtue of epistemic humility. *Philosophy, Psychiatry and Psychology*, 29(2):121–3. https://doi.org/10.1353/ppp.2022.0022

Power, M. (1999). *The audit society: Rituals of verification*. Oxford: Oxford University Press.

Putnam, H. (2002). *The collapse of the fact/value dichotomy and other essays*. Cambridge, MA: Harvard University Press. https://doi.org/10.2307/j.ctv1pdrpz4

Rawls, J. (1999). *A theory of justice*, revised edn. Oxford: Oxford University Press.

Ray, R., Davis, G. (2021). Cultural competence as new racism: Working as intended? *American Journal of Bioethics*, 21:20–2. https://doi.org/10.1080/15265161.2021.1952338

Rice, S.P.M., Shorey-Fennell, B.R. (2020). Comparing the psychometric properties of common measures of positive and negative emotional experiences: Implications for the assessment of subjective wellbeing. *Journal of Well-Being Assessment*, 4:37–56. https://doi.org/10.1007/s41543-020-00025-1

Ricks, T.N., Abbyad, C., Polinard, E. (2022). Undoing racism and mitigating bias among healthcare professionals: Lessons learned during a systematic review.

Journal of Racial and Ethnic Health Disparities, 9:1990–2000. https://doi.
org/10.1007/s40615-021-01137-x

Roberts, D. (2013). Thick concepts. *Philosophy Compass*, 8(8):677–88. https://
doi.org/10.1111/phc3.12055

Rogers, W. (2020). Moral responsibility in medicine: Where are the boundaries?
The Lancet, 396:373–4. https://doi.org/10.1016/S0140-6736(20)31643-3

Rondini, A.C., Kowalsky, R.H., Waggoner, M.R. (2021). Addressing meso-level
mechanisms of racism in medicine. *American Journal of Bioethics*, 21(2):
66–9. https://doi.org/10.1080/15265161.2020.1861372

Royal College of Physicians (2023). *RCP view on healthcare sustainability
and climate change.* https://www.rcp.ac.uk/media/oiqjvojz/rcp-view-on-
healthcare-sustainability-and-climate-change-final-march-2023-_0-2.pdf
(accessed 8 June 2025).

Sackett, D., Rosenberg, W.M.C., Gray, J.A.M., Richardson, W.S. (1996). Evidence
based medicine: What it is and what it isn't. *BMJ*, 312:71. https://doi.
org/10.1136/bmj.312.7023.71

Salisbury, C. (1999). Healthy living centres. *BMJ*, 319:1384–5. https://doi.
org/10.1136/bmj.319.7222.1384

Sayer, A. (2011). *Why things matter to people.* Cambridge: Cambridge University
Press.

Scaccia, J.P., Scott, V.C. (2021). 5335 days of Implementation Science: Using
natural language processing to examine publication trends and topics.
Implementation Science, 16:47. https://doi.org/10.1186/s13012-021-01120-4

Schedler, A. (1999). Conceptualizing accountability. In: Schedler, A.,
Diamond, L.J. and Plattner, M.F. (Eds.), *The self-restraining state: Power and
accountability in new democracies.* Boulder, CO: Lynne Rienner Publishers,
pp. 13–28.

Schulpen, T.W.J., Lombarts, K.M.J. (2007). Quality improvement of paediatric
care in the Netherlands. *Archives of Diseases in Childhood*, 92:633–6. https://
doi.org/10.1136/adc.2006.104091

Seedhouse, D. (1986). *Health: The foundations for achievement.* Chichester:
Wiley.

Sen, A. (1987). *The standard of living.* Cambridge: Cambridge University Press.

Sen, A. (2009). *The idea of justice.* Cambridge, MA: Belknap Press.

Shafer-Landau, R. (Ed.) (2007). *Ethical theory: An anthology.* Oxford: Blackwell
Publishing.

Sheehan, M. (2007). Resources and the rule of rescue. *Journal of Applied
Philosophy*, 24:352–66. https://doi.org/10.1111/j.1468-5930.2007.00383.x

Shewhart, W.A. (1925). The application of statistics as an aid in maintaining
quality of a manufactured product. *Journal of the American Statistical
Association*, 20:546–8. https://doi.org/10.1080/01621459.1925.10502930

Sholl, S., Scheffler, G., Monrouxe, L.V., Rees, C. (2019). Understanding the
healthcare workplace learning culture through safety and dignity narratives:
A UK qualitative study of multiple stakeholders' perspectives. *BMJ Open*,
9:e025615. doi:10.1136/bmjopen-2018-025615

Simpson, R.M. (2013). Dignity, harm, and hate speech. *Law and Philosophy*, 32:701–28. https://doi.org/10.1007/s10982-012-9164-z

Sinclair, S. (2022). Explaining rule of rescue obligations in healthcare allocation: Allowing the patient to tell the right kind of story about their life. *Medicine, Health Care and Philosophy*, 25:31–46. https://doi.org/10.1007/s11019-021-10047-y

Singh, G., Cribb, A. (2021). Aligning quality improvement with better child health for the 21st century. *Archives of Diseases in Childhood – Education and Practice*, 106:370–7. https://doi.org/10.1136/archdischild-2020-318924

Singh, G., Zhu, H. (2020). Poverty in practice: Using quality improvement in paediatrics to improve identification and support of families living in poverty. *Archives of Diseases in Childhood - Education and Practice*, 106:306–9. https://doi.org/10.1136/archdischild-2019-318259

Sliwa, P. (2023). Making sense of things: Moral inquiry as hermeneutical inquiry. *Philosophy and Phenomenological Research*, 109(1):117–37. https://doi.org/10.1111/phpr.13028

Smaggus, A., Goldszmidt, M. (2017). High reliability and 'Cargo Cult QI': Response to Sutcliffe et al. BMJ Qual Saf, 201726:248–51. *BMJ Quality & Safety*, 26:518. https://doi.org/10.1136/bmjqs-2017-006748

Snow, C.P. [1959] (2012). *The two cultures*. Cambridge: Cambridge University Press.

Sokol-Hessner, L., Folcarelli, P.H., Sands, K.E.F. (2015). Emotional harm from disrespect: The neglected preventable harm. *BMJ Quality & Safety*, 24:550–3. https://doi.org/10.1136/bmjqs-2015-004034

Star, S.L., Griesemer, J.R. (1989). Institutional ecology, 'translations' and boundary objects: Amateurs and professionals in Berkeley's Museum of Vertebrate Zoology, 1907–39. *Social Studies of Science*, 19(3):387–420. https://doi.org/10.1177/030631289019003001

Stewart, M.A., Brown, J.B., Weston, W., McWhinney, I.R., McWilliam, C.L., Freeman, T. (2013). *Patient-centered medicine: Transforming the clinical method*, 3rd edn. Boca Raton, FL: CRC Press.

Sun, G.H., MacEachern, M.P., Perla, R.J., Gaines, J.M., Davis, M.M., Shrank, W.H. (2014). Health care quality improvement publication trends. *American Journal of Medical Quality*, 29(5):403–7. https://doi.org/10.1177/1062860613503708

The Health Foundation (2024). *The contribution of the health and care system to improving health*. https://www.health.org.uk/what-we-do/supporting-health-care-improvement/the-contribution-of-the-health-and-care-system-to-improving-health (accessed 30 April 2024).

The Health Foundation (n.d.). *Supporting radical innovation and improvement in health and care services*. https://www.health.org.uk/strategic-priorities/supporting-innovation-in-health-and-care-services (accessed 31 May 2025).

The Royal College of Surgeons of England (n.d.). *Surgical outcomes: Driving up standards of care for patients through publishing surgeons outcomes data*. https://www.rcseng.ac.uk/patient-care/surgical-staff-and-regulation/surgical-outcomes/ (accessed 16 June 2025).

Thiele, L.P. (2024). *Sustainability*, 3rd edn. Cambridge: Polity Press.

Thomas, E.J. (2020). The harms of promoting 'Zero Harm'. *BMJ Quality & Safety*, 29:4–6. https://doi.org/10.1136/bmjqs-2019-009703

Thomas, J.M., Cosford, P.A. (2010). Place sustainability at the heart of the quality agenda. *Quality and Safety in Health Care*, 19(4):260–1. https://doi.org/10.1136/qshc.2010.044123

UK Government (2012). Health and Social Care Act 2012. https://www.legislation.gov.uk/ukpga/2012/7/contents/enacted (accessed 11 January 2026).

UK National Screening Committee (2022). *Guidance: Criteria for a population screening programme*. https://www.gov.uk/government/publications/evidence-review-criteria-national-screening-programmes/criteria-for-appraising-the-viability-effectiveness-and-appropriateness-of-a-screening-programme (accessed 9 June 2025).

University of Washington (2023). *Where to start? There are so many!* https://impsciuw.org/implementation-science/research/frameworks/ (accessed 9 June 2025).

Valles, S.A. (2018). *Philosophy of population health: Philosophy for a new public health era*. London: Routledge.

Venkatapuram, S. (2011). *Health justice: An argument from the capabilities approach*. Cambridge: Polity.

Vincent, C., Burnett, S., Carthey, J. (2014). Safety measurement and monitoring in healthcare: A framework to guide clinical teams and healthcare organisations in maintaining safety. *BMJ Quality & Safety*, 23(8):670–7. https://doi.org/10.1136/bmjqs-2013-002757

Weale, A. (2011). New modes of governance, political accountability and public reason. *Government and Opposition*, 46(1):58–80. https://doi.org/10.1111/j.1477-7053.2010.01330.x

WHAM Project (n.d.). WHAM Project. https://www.whamproject.co.uk/ (accessed 22 November 2023).

Wilegoda, M., Gupta, C., Khattak, J., Aidoo-Micah, G., Chowdhury, L. (2016). G568(P) Standardisation of paediatric handovers – a quality improvement project. *Archives of Disease in Childhood*, 101(S1):A338. https://doi.org/10.1136/archdischild-2016-310863.554

Wilfond, B.S., Ravitsky, V. (2005). On the proliferation of bioethics sub-disciplines: Do we really need 'Genethics' and 'Neuroethics'? *American Journal of Bioethics*, 5(2):20–1. https://doi.org/10.1080/15265160590960924

Wilson, J., Hunter, D. (2010). Research exceptionalism. *American Journal of Bioethics*, 10(8):45–54. https://doi.org/10.1080/15265161.2010.482630

Wilson, J., Jungner, G. (1968). *Principles and practice of screening for disease*. Public Health Papers No. 34. Geneva: World Health Organization.

Wittgenstein, L. (1986). *Philosophical investigations*, 3rd edn. Oxford: Blackwell.

Wolff, J. (2019). *Ethics and public policy: A philosophical inquiry*, 2nd edn. Abingdon: Routledge. https://doi.org/10.4324/9781351128667

World Health Organization (2018). *Handbook for national quality policy and strategy: A practical approach for developing policy and strategy to improve quality of care.* Geneva: World Health Organization.

Young, I.M. (1990). *Justice and the politics of difference.* Princeton, NJ: Princeton University Press.

Young, I.M. (2001). Equality of whom? Social groups and judgments of injustice. *Journal of Political Philosophy*, 9(1):1–18. https://doi.org/10.1111/1467-9760.00115